简明汉英中医养生词典

Concise Chinese-English Dictionary of Health Preservation in Traditional Chinese Medicine

主审◎陈　锋

主编◎方廷钰　张清怡　刘　平

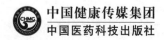
中国健康传媒集团
中国医药科技出版社

内 容 提 要

　　本词典收录中医养生基本字、词、术语、概念和经典用语1万余条。作者根据近年来出版的中外中医辞书和中医药翻译的最新进展，并结合自己长期以来的翻译经验和研究体会，对古奥玄秘的中医养生用语进行了深入的研究分析，明确其语义内涵，编纂成此词典。本词典不仅提供了中医养生词条的英语对应词，还提供了例语和例句，可供中医院校师生、中医药工作者、中西医结合工作者、中医英语翻译工作者及其他相关领域研究人员参阅。

图书在版编目（CIP）数据

　　简明汉英中医养生词典/方廷钰，张清怡，刘平主编 . —北京：中国医药科技出版社，2024.1

　　ISBN 978 - 7 - 5214 - 4123 - 9

　　Ⅰ.①简… 　Ⅱ.①方…②张…③刘… 　Ⅲ.①养生（中医）—词典—汉、英 　Ⅳ.①R212 - 61

　　中国国家版本馆 CIP 数据核字（2023）第 161765 号

美术编辑　陈君杞
版式设计　诚达誉高

出版　**中国健康传媒集团** ｜ 中国医药科技出版社
地址　北京市海淀区文慧园北路甲 22 号
邮编　100082
电话　发行：010 - 62227427　邮购：010 - 62236938
网址　www. cmstp. com
规格　880×1230mm ½₃₂
印张　9⅝
字数　367 千字
版次　2024 年 1 月第 1 版
印次　2024 年 1 月第 1 次印刷
印刷　北京盛通印刷股份有限公司
经销　全国各地新华书店
书号　ISBN 978 - 7 - 5214 - 4123 - 9
定价　**88.00 元**

获取新书信息、投稿、为图书纠错，请扫码联系我们。

编 委 会

前　言

中医药作为中华文明的杰出代表，是中华文化走向世界的重要内容。习近平总书记在中央政治局第三十次集体学习时强调："要更好推动中华文化走出去，以文载道、以文传声、以文化人，向世界阐释推介更多具有中国特色、体现中国精神、蕴藏中国智慧的优秀文化。"精准的中医翻译会助力中医更好地"走出去"。

目前，中外学者已出版了多部汉英中医学词典，但尚未见以中医养生为主题的汉英词典，为填补这一空白，五年前我们即着手编写汉英中医养生词典，由于中途受到疫情影响，直至近期才终于完成了全书的编写和审阅工作。

本书作为一部中医养生词典，除中医基础、生理、病理及临床相关词目外，还提供了大量《黄帝内经》以及诸子百家著作中的养生经文。例如："所以能年皆度百岁而动作不衰者，以其德全不危也。They all lived over one hundred years without any signs of senility because they could follow the tenets of preserving health. "（《素问·上古天真论》）；"生而勿杀，予而勿夺，赏而勿罚，此春气之应，养生之道也。Promote growth instead of destruction, give more and take less, reward more and punish less. This is in accordance with the principle of springtime to nurture and it is the way to keep fit. "（《素问·四气调神大论》）；"仁者寿 long life enjoyed by benevolent people"（《论语·雍也》）；"八不食 eight forbidden rules in eating"（《论语·乡党》）；"道法自然 divine law following nature"（《道德经》）；"清净无为 being quiet and having fewer desires"（《虑子贱碑颂》）；"少不勤行，壮不竞时，长而安贫……养生之方也。A person is neither excessively fond of having a good time in childhood nor seeking instant success and quick profits when young, and he is happy to live a simple life in middle age... This is the sound strategy for health preservation." (《列子》)；"坐忘、心斋 seating in oblivion and purifying the mind"(《庄子》)；"养生常欲小劳，但莫大疲及强所不能堪耳。To keep fit, it is necessary to do a little physical labor to the extent that one can tolerate." (《备急千金要方》)；"田夫寿，膏粱夭。Farmers usually enjoy a long life while wealthy people die young." (《养性延命录》)。在新型冠状病毒肺炎疫情背景下，本书中也收录了《礼记·月令》"孟春行秋令，则民大疫。If in the first month of spring there is autumn-like weather, pandemic will prevail." 等疫病相关经文。

　　同时，书中还包含情志养生、饮食养生、起居养生、运动养生等方面内容。全书共收录四千余词目和两千余例语、例句，在一半的词目下附有例语和例句，有助于读者查阅中医术语英译的同时也了解中医语句的翻译方法，以便举一反三，掌握中医翻译技巧。本书中医术语、典籍经文译文以信为本，力求与时俱进、有所创新，修正误读误译，为中医英译探索新的途径，希望得到社会认可。

　　书后附有中英对照的养生相关典籍、养生相关中药 2 个附录，译文不尽完美，供读者参考。编写工作中难免存有疏漏，敬请广大读者不吝赐教，提出宝贵意见，以便再版时修正。

方廷钰
于北京中医药大学
2023 年 4 月 20 日

凡　例

一、本词典分为正文和附录两部分。

二、正文以汉语词目第一个字的汉语拼音顺序排列，并以四声为序。

三、本词典的词目内容按汉语词目、汉语拼音、英语释义、例语和例句顺序排列。

四、一般情况下每个汉语词目对应一个英语词，有两个及以上对应词时，用"，"隔开。例如："本质 essence, nature"。

五、汉语词目多义时，英语对应词用"；"隔开。例如："露 distillate; syrup; juice"，"安心 being at ease; setting one's mind on"。

六、汉语词目为句子时，英语词以短语或句子的形式出现。例如："白头偕老 living to a ripe old age in conjugal bliss"，"百废俱兴 All that was left undone is now being restarted"。

七、正文内中药名一律使用汉语拼音加英文名称，拉丁文仅在附录中出现。

八、为保持规范英语，英语定冠词、不定冠词和介词一律不省略。

目　　录

检 字 表

A

A

阿 A

阿 ā

阿是穴［ā shì xué］*Ashi* acupoint 以痛为俞，治取 ~。An *Ashi* acupoint located at the tender spot is selected.

哀埃嗳艾爱 AI

哀 āi

哀［āi］sorrow, sympathy ~悼 mourning/ ~乐 dirge/ ~而不伤 being mourning but not sad

埃 āi

埃昏［āi hūn］spread of dust ~布作 spread of dust in the sky

埃雾［āi wù］dust and fog ~蒙郁 heavy dust, fog and miasma

埃云［āi yún］dust like fog ~润泽 Dust swirls in the air with gentle breeze and drizzle.

埃骤［āi zhòu］a lot of dust and heavey rain ~注之变 sudden attack by heavy dust and rain

嗳 ǎi

嗳腐［ǎi fǔ］putrid belching ~吞酸 putrid belching and swallowing upcast gastric acid

嗳 ài

嗳气［ài qì］belching

艾 ài

艾［ài］argy wormwood leaf ~卷 moxa roll ~卷灸 moxa-roll moxibustion

艾灸［ài jiǔ］moxibustion ~补泻 reinforcing and reducing method in moxibustion/ ~包括艾条灸、太乙神针和雷火神针。Moxibustion includes moxibustion with moxa stick, *Taiyi*-miraculous moxa stick and thunder-fire miraculous moxa stick.

艾绒［ài róng］wormwood floss 纯净细软的 ~ fine, soft wormwood floss

艾叶［ài yè］argy wormwood leaf ~炭 carbonized argy wormwood leaves/ ~气味芳香。A sweet fragrance rises from argy wormwood leaves. / ~性温，行气活血，温经散寒。Argy wormwood leaf, warm in property, works to promote qi and blood circulation, warm meridians and dissipate cold.

爱 ài

爱［ài］love 她对《红楼梦》~不释手。She loves *A Dream of Red Mansion* so much that she cannot stop reading it.

爱巢［ài cháo］love nest

A

爱抚[ài fǔ] having tender affection for

爱河[ài hé] river of love 坠入 ~ falling in love

爱护[ài hù] taking good care of 相互 ~ care about each other

爱恋[ài liàn] being in love with ~ 之情 loving feelings

爱美[ài měi] being particular about one's appearance; loving beautiful things ~ 之心，人皆有之。Loving beauty is one part of human nature.

爱屋及乌[ài wū jí wū] Love me, love my dog.

爱心[ài xīn] affection 献 ~ extending compassion/充满 ~ full of love

爱憎分明[ài zēng fēn míng] being clear about what or who to love or hate

安按案暗 AN
安 ān

安不忘危[ān bù wàng wēi] being mindful of potential danger during times of peace

安常处顺[ān cháng chǔ shùn] taking things as they are

安定[ān dìng] stable ~ 情绪 stabilizing one's emotions/ ~ 团结 stability and unity/过 ~ 的生活 leading a stable life

安度[ān dù] spending peacefully ~ 难关 tiding over difficulties/ ~ 晚年 living out one's final years in peace

安顿[ān dùn] making proper arrangements 先把病人 ~ 好。Help the patient to settle down first.

安分[ān fèn] knowing one's place ~ 守己。Know one's place and mind one's own business.

安抚[ān fǔ] appeasing ~ 民心 reassuring and appeasing the popular feelings

安家[ān jiā] setting up a home ~ 落户 setting down

安居处[ān jū chù] maintaining regular daily life

安居乐业[ān jū lè yè] living in prosperity and contentment

安康[ān kāng] good health

安乐[ān lè] peace and happiness 过 ~ 的生活 leading a peaceful and happy life/ ~ 死 euthanasia

安眠[ān mián] sleeping peacefully ~ 疗法 sleep therapy/ ~ 药 sleeping pills

安民告示[ān mín gào shì] notice to reassure the public; advanced notice

安宁[ān níng] peacefulness; calmness 心里很不 ~ feeling rather worried

安其居[ān qí jū] living in peace and comfort

安寝[ān qǐn] sleeping peacefully ~ 须以清心为要。A clear mind is the key to a peaceful sleep.

安全[ān quán] safety ~ 感 sense of security/人身 ~ personal safety

安然自愉[ān rán zì yú] taking the rough with the smooth 有时还得学会 ~ 。One sometimes must learn to take

A

the rough with the smooth.

安身［ān shēn］taking shelter ~立命 settling down and getting on with one's life/ ~之地 a place to stay

安神［ān shén］calming (anchoring) the mind ~定志 calming the mind/ ~药 mind-calming medicinals

安适［ān shì］quiet and comfortable ~的生活 quiet and comfortable life

安闲［ān xián］leisurely ~自在 leisurely and carefree

安心［ān xīn］being at ease; setting one's mind on ~定气 calming the mind and keeping smooth flow of qi/ ~学习 setting one's mind on study

安逸［ān yì］easy and comfortable 他退休后过着 ~的生活。After retirement he enjoyed an easy and comfortable life.

安枕无忧［ān zhěn wú yōu］rest assured without anxiety

安之若素［ān zhī ruò sù］bearing hardship with equanimity

按 àn

按法［àn fǎ］pressing 掌 ~ palm pressing/指 ~ finger pressing/肘 ~ elbow pressing

按积［àn jī］treating abdominal mass with pressing manipulations ~抑痹 treating abdominal mass with pressure to prevent impediment

按脉［àn mài］taking pulse; pressing meridians ~动静 taking pulse to sense its changes/ ~取气, 令邪出 pressing meridians to drive pathogenic factors out of the body

按摩［àn mó］massage ~醪药 massage with medicated liquor

按目运气［àn mù yùn qì］pressing eyes to guide qi ~可以助眠。Pressing eyes to guide qi helps to fall asleep.

按跷［àn qiāo］ancient term for *tuina*-massage

按双眉［àn shuāng méi］massage applied to brows

按压［àn yā］pressure-massage ~痛甚者为实证 It is an excess pattern when pain aggravates on pressing.

按诊［àn zhěn］body palpation

按之内痛［àn zhī nèi tòng］abdominal pain when pressing

按之痛止［àn zhī tòng zhǐ］relief of pain when pressing

按之至骨［àn zhī zhì gǔ］pressing the pulse deep upon the radius

案 àn

案扤［àn wù］*tuina*-massage

暗 àn

暗经［àn jīng］latent menstruation ~者, 终生不来月经, 但有怀孕的可能。A woman with latent menstruation or life-long absence of menstruation has the potential for pregnancy.

熬懊 AO

熬 áo

熬［áo］cooking in water, boiling,

B

stewing ~膏服 boiling it down into an extract for oral taking/ ~药 boiling medicinal herbs

熬夜[áo yè] staying up late ~是不良习惯,容易缺乏内源氧。Staying up late is a bad habit, which may easily cause a lack of endogenous oxygen. / ~时,应时时做深长呼吸。We should often do deep breathing when staying up late.

熬粥[áo zhōu] cooking congee

懊 ào

懊热[ào rè] vexing fever

B

八拔 BA

八 bā

八宝[bā bǎo] eight treasures ~菜 eight-treasure pickles/ ~饭 eight-treasure rice pudding/ ~箱 treasure box/ ~粥 eight-treasure rice congee

八不食[bā bù shí] eight forbidden rules in eating ~是儒家的教诲。The eight forbidden rules in eating are Confucian teachings.

八段锦[bā duàn jǐn] eight-section brocade 坐式 ~ sitting-styled eight-section brocade/立式 ~ standing-styled eight-section brocade

八风[bā fēng] wind from eight directions; name of acupoint (EX-LE)

八纲辨证[bā gāng biàn zhèng] differentiation of patterns according to the eight principles ~以阴阳为总纲。Yin and yang are the leading factors in pattern differentiation according to the theory of eight principles.

八会穴[bā huì xué] eight influential acupoints ~分布在躯干部和四肢部。The eight influential acupoints are on the trunk and four limbs.

八纪[bā jì] eight solar terms: Beginning of Spring, Spring Equinox, Beginning of Summer, Summer Solstice, Beginning of Autumn, Autumn Equinox, Beginning of Winter and Winter Solstice

八节[bā jié] eight joints (located at the elbow, wrist, knee and ankle)

八脉交会穴[bā mài jiāo huì xué] eight confluence acupoints ~分布于腕踝关节的上下。The eight confluence acupoints are located above or below the wrists and ankle joints.

八珍[bā zhēn] eight delicacies

八正[bā zhèng] eight solar terms; eight directions

B

八字[bā zì] Eight Chinese Characters 生辰 ~ Eight Chinese Characters used to tell one's time, date of birth

拔 bá

拔背[bá bèi] keeping the trunk erect

拔毒 [bá dú] drawing out toxic substances 火罐 ~ drawing out toxic substances with cupping/ ~ 法 method of drawing out toxic substances/ ~ 膏 toxic substance removing plaster

拔罐[bá guàn] cupping ~疗法 cupping therapy/刺血 ~ 法 blood-letting and cupping/留针 ~ 法 needle-retainingcupping/寒湿背痛,可采用 ~ 方法。The cupping therapy is adopted for back pain due to cold and dampness.

拔脓 [bá nóng] draining pus ~ 毒 draining pus and toxic substances/ ~ 解毒 draining pus to expel toxic substances/ ~ 托腐 draining pus to remove putrefaction

拔伸法[bá shēn fǎ] traction therapy 颈部 ~ traction of the neck/肩关节 ~ traction of the shoulder joint/指关节 ~ traction of the interphalangeal joint

拔丝[bá sī] caramelizing ~ 山药 toffee yam

拔针[bá zhēn] withdrawing a needle

拔直捏正[bá zhí niē zhèng] reduction by pulling and kneading

白百摆败拜 BAI
白 bái

白案[bái àn] flour or rice cooking

白茶[bái chá] white tea ~ 淡雅清香, 滋润人的肺腑。White tea with wafts of sweet scent provides nourishment to the lung.

白癜风[bái diàn fēng] vitiligo

白喉 [bái hóu] diphtheria ~ 三不可 three forbidden things in treatment for diphtheria

白芥子灸 [bái jiè zǐ jiǔ] Baijiezi (Mustard Seed) moxibustion

白睛 [bái jīng] the white of eyes, bulbar conjunctiva ~ 红赤 redness of the white of eyes/ ~ 涩痛 irritant and painful bulbar conjunctiva/ ~ 萎黄 conjunctival xanthosis/ ~ 溢血 subconjunctival ecchymosis

白酒[bái jiǔ] liquor, spirit

白开水 [bái kāi shuǐ] plain boiled water

白里透红 [bái lǐ tòu hóng] white complexion with rosy color

白露[bái lù] White Dew

白木耳[bái mù ěr] edible white fungus

白内障[bái nèi zhàng] cataract ~针拨 术 cataractopiesis with a metal needle

白肉[bái ròu] white meat; plain boiled pork; the meat on the inside of the thigh

白如枯骨[bái rú kū gǔ] countenance as white as dry bones ~ 者死。The countenance as white as dry bones is a fatal sign.

白色污染 [bái sè wū rǎn] white pollution from plastic bags, etc.

B

白砂苔[bái shā tāi] white sandy fur

白糖[bái táng] white sugar

白天[bái tiān] in the daytime, during the day ～的气温 temperature in the daytime

白头偕老[bái tóu xié lǎo] living to a ripe old age in conjugal bliss

白翳[bái yì] nebula

白昼[bái zhòu] daytime

百 bǎi

百病[bǎi bìng] all kinds of diseases ～多由痰作祟。 All kinds of diseases are triggered by phlegm.

百病生于气[bǎi bìng shēng yú qì] All diseases result from qi disorder. 凡表里虚实，逆顺缓急，无不因气而至，故 ～。 Qi disorder may lead to any pattern, whether exterior, interior, deficiency, excess, or any other conditions, whether deteriorative, favorable, chronic or acute. That is why to say "all diseases result from qi disorder".

百草[bǎi cǎo] all kinds of herbs 神农尝 ～， 始有医药。 The birth of traditional Chinese medicine was when Shen Nong tasted hundreds of herbs.

百废俱兴[bǎi fèi jù xīng] All that was left undone is now being restarted.

百感交集[bǎi gǎn jiāo jí] All sorts of feelings well up in one's heart.

百骸[bǎi hái] limbs and skeleton

百合病[bǎi hé bìng] diseases which can be treated with *Baihe* (lily) and related formula

百疾[bǎi jí] all diseases ～之始期也，必生于风雨寒暑。 Occurrence of all diseases is exclusively caused by wind, rain, cold and summer-heat.

百酱[bǎi jiàng] various seasonings

百节[bǎi jié] joints of the body ～尽皆纵 looseness of all joints

百科全书[bǎi kē quán shū] encyclopedia

百里挑一[bǎi lǐ tiāo yī] one in a hundred, the cream of the crop 他的医术就是好，可谓 ～。 What a good doctor he is, the cream of the crop, so to speak.

百炼成钢[bǎi liàn chéng gāng] being tempered into steel

百年[bǎi nián] one hundred years old ～不衰 enduring for one hundred years/ ～之好 remaining a devoted couple to the end of their lives

百日咳[bǎi rì ké] whooping cough

百岁[bǎi suì] a life span of one hundred years ～老人 centenarian/所以能年皆度 ～而动作不衰者，以其德全不危也。 They all lived over one hundred years without any signs of senility because they could follow the tenets of preserving health.

百无禁忌[bǎi wú jìn jì] no restrictions of any kind

百无聊赖[bǎi wú liáo lài] being bored to death

百无一失[bǎi wú yī shī] no risk at all

百馐[bǎi xiū] various delicacies

百药 [bǎi yào] various kinds of medicinals

百叶包 [bǎi yè bāo] stuffed roll (wrapped with thin sheets of bean curd)

摆 bǎi

摆件[bǎi jiàn] ornaments

摆酒[bǎi jiǔ] giving a feast

败 bài

败火[bài huǒ] relieving internal heat

拜 bài

拜佛[bài fó] worshiping Buddha 烧香 ~ burning incense and worshipping Buddha

癍瘢扳斑半 BAN

癍 bān

癍[bān] fleck

瘢 bān

瘢[bān] scar ~ 痕 scar

扳 bān

扳法 [bān fǎ] pulling 颈椎 ~ pulling the cervical vertebrae/胸背部 ~ pulling the chest and back/腰部 ~ pulling the lower back

扳腿手法[bān tuǐ shǒu fǎ] leg-pulling manipulation

斑 bān

斑秃[bān tū] alopecia areata

斑疹[bān zhěn] macula ~ 伤寒 typhus/ ~ 稀疏 sparse macular eruptions/ ~ 隐现 macular eruptions occurring now

and then

半 bàn

半百 [bàn bǎi] 50 years old ~ 而衰 senilism at 50 years old

半辈子[bàn bèi zi] half a lifetime 大 ~ the greater part of one's life/上 ~ the first half of one's life

半表半里证 [bàn biǎo bàn lǐ zhèng] half-exterior and half-interior pattern

半刺[bàn cì] shallow puncturing ~ 者，浅内而疾发针、无针伤肉。Shallow puncturing refers to inserting a needle superficially and withdrawing it quickly without injury to the muscle.

半发酵茶 [bàn fā jiào chá] semi-fermented tea 长期饮用 ~ 对人体有很好的保健作用。Long-term drinking of semi-fermented tea is good for health.

半流食[bàn liú shí] semi-liquid diet

半身 [bàn shēn] half body ~ 不遂 hemiplegia/ ~ 汗出 hemihyperidrosis/ ~ 麻木 hemianesthesia/ ~ 无汗 half-body absence of sweating

半生不熟 [bàn shēng bù shú] half-cooked

半夜 [bàn yè] midnight ~ 三更 in the depth of night/下 ~ after midnight

帮傍 BANG

帮 bāng

帮厨[bāng chú] being a kitchen help

傍 bàng

傍针刺[bàng zhēn cì] straight and side

B

needling ~ 者,直刺旁刺各一,以治留痹久居者也。In treatment for chronic arthralgia two needles inserted perpendicularly and obliquely into the affected part is known as the straight and side needling.

胞煲雹薄饱保葆报抱暴 BAO
胞 bāo

胞宫[bāo gōng] womb, uterus ~ 主月经,主孕育胎儿。The uterus is responsible for menstruation discharge, pregnancy and development of fetus.

胞络[bāo luò] uterine collateral ~ 空虚 deficiency in the uterine collateral/ ~ 伤而下崩 metrorrhagia due to injury to the uterine collateral

胞脉[bāo mài] uterine vessel ~ 不通 obstruction of the uterine vessel/ ~ 受损 impairment of the uterine vessel/ ~ 的主要作用是主女子月经和妊育胞胎。The uterine vessel is responsible for menstruation, pregnancy and development of fetus. / 月事不来, ~ 闭也。Amenorrhea is due to obstruction of the uterine vessel. / ~ 者,属心而络于胞中。The uterine vessel attributes to the heart and connects with the uterus.

胞门[bāo mén] ostium of the uterus 产后 ~ 不闭 unclosure of the ostium of the uterus after childbirth

胞衣[bāo yī] placenta ~ 不下 placenta retention after childbirth

煲 bāo

煲汤[bāo tāng] casserole soup

雹 báo

雹[báo] hailstone

薄 báo

薄白苔[báo bái tāi] thin and white coating

薄饼[báo bǐng] thin pancake

薄唇[báo chún] thin lips ~ 轻言 being gossipy/不干你的事,别 ~ 轻言。It's none of your business, keep your mouth shut. /玛丽是个 ~ 轻言的人。Mary is a great one for idle gossip.

薄脆饼[báo cuì bǐng] crisp fritter

薄皮[báo pí] white complexion ~ 弱肉 people with white complexion, thin skin and weak muscles

薄苔[báo tāi] thin fur, thin coating

薄药[báo yào] herbal medicinals bland in taste and mild in nature

饱 bǎo

饱餐[bǎo cān] eating one's fill ~ 一顿 eating a big meal

饱经风霜[bǎo jīng fēng shuāng] having the experienced hardships of life, weather-beaten

保 bǎo

保健[bǎo jiàn] health and fitness, health care ~ 按摩 health care massage/ ~ 操 health exercises/ ~ 食品 health food/ ~ 用品 health product/妇幼 ~ health care for women and children/全民 ~ public health work/日常 ~daily health maintenance

保健功[bǎo jiàn gōng] fitness *qigong* ~可以活动筋骨,促进血液循环。Fitness *qigong* helps promote joint movement and blood circulation.

保暖[bǎo nuǎn] keeping warm 足浴可以改善脚部的血液流动,有利于 ~。Foot bath works to promote foot blood circulation, which ensures keeping warm.

保气[bǎo qì] preserving qi ~ 养神 preserving qi to repose/~ 存精 preserving qi and essence

保湿[bǎo shī] retaining moisture ~ 唇膏 moisturizing lipstick/~ 护肤 skin moisturizer/~ 面霜 face-moisturizing cream/~ 摩丝 moisturizing mousse/有助于皮肤 ~ helping to moisturize the skin

保胎[bǎo tāi] preventing miscarriage

保温[bǎo wēn] heat preservation; keeping warm ~杯 vacuum cup

保鲜[bǎo xiān] keeping something fresh ~ 袋 fresh-keeping bag/~ 膜 fresh-keeping film

保胃气[bǎo wèi qì] preserving stomach-qi ~,养胃阴 preserving stomach-qi and replenishing stomach-yin

保形全神[bǎo xíng quán shén] keeping the physique and structure of the body and spirit well

保养[bǎo yǎng] taking good care of 皮肤 ~ skin care

保质期[bǎo zhì qī] best before..., exp. date ~ 至 2020 年 9 月 best before Sep. 2020, Exp. 09/2020

葆 bǎo

葆[bǎo] preserving 永 ~ 青春 preserving one's youthful look

报 bào

报刺[bào cì] successive trigger needling ~ 者,刺痛无常处也。Successive trigger needling refers to acupuncture applied directly to a tender spot, and then search for other tender spots over the surrounding area and acupuncture is applied again.

抱 bào

抱头火丹[bào tóu huǒ dān] head or facial erysipelas

暴 bào

暴痹[bào bì] sudden occurrence of impediment

暴病[bào bìng] sudden attack by a serious disease ~ 猝死 sudden death due to severe illness

暴厥[bào jué] sudden syncope ~ 而聋 deafness due to sudden syncope

暴乐暴苦[bào lè bào kǔ] violent anger and overjoy

暴聋[bào lóng] sudden deafness

暴盲[bào máng] sudden blindness

暴怒[bào nù] sudden rage ~ 伤阴 Sudden rage damages yin.

暴仆[bào pū] sudden loss of consciousness

暴热[bào rè] sudden high fever (usually seen in an excess-heat pattern）

暴食［bào shí］overeating ～不节 gorging oneself, taking excessive improper food/暴饮 ～ overdrinking and overeating/暴饮 ～ 损害健康。Excess at table injures health.

暴殄天物［bào tiǎn tiān wù］reckless waste of products of nature

暴痛［bào tòng］sudden pain

暴亡［bào wáng］sudden death

暴袭［bào xí］sudden assailing ～气蒙 dizziness with blurred vision due to sudden attack by pathogenic factors

暴瘖［bào yīn］sudden aphonia

暴躁［bào zào］irritable 脾气 ～ being hot-tempered

暴注［bào zhù］sudden severe diarrhea

暴卒［bào zú］sudden death

悲背 BEI
悲 bēi

悲哀［bēi āi］grieved, sad ～的心情 sad feeling/ ～ 愁忧 sorrow, grief, worry and anxious/ ～ 动中。Excessive sorrow and grief disturb the internal. / ～愁忧则心动,心动则五脏六腑皆摇。Grief and worry cause heart disturbance, and eventually affects the zang-fu organs.

悲欢离合［bēi huān lí hé］joys and sorrows 人有 ～ People may suffer from joys and sorrows.

悲伤［bēi shāng］sorrow ～ 不乐 sorrowful and unhappy

悲胜怒［bēi shèng nù］anger overcomed by grief

悲喜交集［bēi xǐ jiāo jí］mixed feeling of grief and joy

悲则气消［bēi zé qì xiāo］qi consumption due to great sadness

悲壮［bēi zhuàng］solemn and stirring

背 bēi

背法［bēi fǎ］back to back carrying therapy

背 bèi

背风［bèi fēng］leeward ～而居 living protected from the wind/在房屋 ～ 的一处 in the leeward of the house

背光［bèi guāng］badly-lit

背强［bèi jiàng］stiff back

背瞀［bèi mào］oppression in the back ～胸满 oppression in the back with stuffiness in the chest

背俞穴［bèi shù xué］back transport acupoint

背腧中背［bèi shù zhòng bèi］To treat disorders of the yang meridians, the acupoints located on the back should be selected.

背宜常暖［bèi yí cháng nuǎn］constantly keeping the back warm 风寒之邪极易通过背部侵入,损伤阳气,故 ～。Wind-cold easily invades the back and impairs yang-qi, so we should constantly keep the back warm.

背阴[bèi yīn] shady 楼后的 ~ 地方 in the shade of the building

背膺[bèi yīng] back and chest ~ 厚者，肺端正。Thicker back and chest indicates that the lung is uprightly located.

奔本 BEN

奔 bēn

奔豚气[bēn tún qì] sensation of piglet running

本 běn

本[běn] origin, root cause; body resistance ~ 寒标热 cold in nature and hot in superficiality/ ~ 虚标实 deficiency in nature and excess in superficiality/病为 ~，工为标，标本不得，邪气不服，此之谓也。A patient is the root, and a doctor is the branch. If there is a lack of coordination between the root and the branch, it would be difficult to suppress the pathogens even if the doctor is brilliant.

本草[běn cǎo] materia medica

本经配穴法[běn jīng pèi xué fǎ] acupoint combination of the same meridian

本能[běn néng] instinct

本性[běn xìng] natural instincts

本质[běn zhì] essence, nature 透过现象看 ~ seeing through the appearance to the essence

崩绷蹦 BENG

崩 bēng

崩漏[bēng lòu] abnormal uterine bleeding, metrorrhagia or metrostaxis

绷 bēng

绷带[bēng dài] bandage

蹦 bèng

蹦床[bèng chuáng] trampoline

鼻比闭辟避臂痹 BI

鼻 bí

鼻[bí] nose ~ 孔 nostrils/ ~ 尖 tip of the nose/ ~ 疳 nasal eczema

鼻不闻香臭[bí bù wén xiāng chòu] loss of smell

鼻槁[bí gǎo] dry nose

鼻鼾[bí hān] snore ~ 声重 loud snores

鼻流清涕[bí liú qīng tì] runny nose with clear thin discharge

鼻衄[bí nù] nose bleeding, epistaxis

鼻鼽[bí qiú] allergic rhinitis

鼻塞[bí sè] nasal congestion ~ 声重 low muffled voice/ ~ 不利少气 stuffy nose with shortness of breath

鼻煽[bí shān] flaring of nares 肺气不利，呼吸急促， ~ 不止。Impeded lung-qi results in shortness of breath and flaring of nares.

鼻吸口呼[bí xī kǒu hū] nasal breathing in and oral breathing out

鼻渊[bí yuān] sinusitis

鼻针[bí zhēn] nose acupuncture ~ 疗法 nose acupuncture therapy/ ~ 麻醉 nose

B

B

acupuncture anesthesia

鼻痔[bí zhì] nasal polyp

比 bǐ

比类取象 [bǐ lèi qǔ xiàng] corresponding resonance understood through analogy

闭 bì

闭藏[bì cáng] storage 冬三月,此谓～。 During the three months of winter, the vitality of all things on earth is hidden.

闭经[bì jīng] amenorrhea 生理性～ physiological amenorrhea/病理性～ pathological amenorrhea/冲任不足, 月经失调,甚则～。Deficiency in the Thoroughfare Vessel and Conception Vessel results in menstural irregularity,even amenorrhea.

闭目养神[bì mù yǎng shén] closing eyes in repose ～是我国先民养神修性的一种简便易行的方法。Chinese ancestors used to sit and relax with eyes closed to cultivate themselves. / ～是最简单的养肝之法。Closing one's eyes in repose is the easiest way to nourish the liver.

闭气[bì qì] holding breath ～ 不息 holding breath/～是通过特殊的呼吸方法达到养生的目的。Holding breath is a special way of breathing, which is good for health.

闭塞 [bì sè] obstruction ～ 不通 obstruction/～ 而不行 obstruction of qi due to invasion by pathogenic factors

闭药 [bì yào] medicinals for breaking obstruction

闭证[bì zhèng] block pattern in stroke

辟 bì

辟谷[bì gǔ] fasting ～在西汉时期很流行。Fasting is in vogue in the Western Han Dynasty (206 B. C. – 24 A. D.) in China.

辟秽[bì huì] exorcising foul matter 芳香～法 exorcising filth with aromatics

避 bì

避风 [bì fēng] parrying wind ～ 防冻 taking shelter from the wind and preventing frostbite/～ 如避箭。Parrying wind is just like parrying arrows. /四时惟夏难调理,夏夜～如避矢。It is most difficult to nurse one's health in summer because it is not easy to parry wind on summer night just like to parry arrows.

避年[bì nián] annual menstruation

避暑 [bì shǔ] avoiding summer-heat; preventing sunstroke

避邪[bì xié] exorcising evil spirits

臂 bì

臂[bì] arm ～内廉 medial arm

臂内[bì nèi] medial aspect of the arm

臂肘[bì zhǒu] elbow ～挛急 spasm of the elbow

痹 bì

痹[bì] impediment; blockage of qi and blood/ ～证 impediment pattern/行 ～ migratory arthralgia/着 ～ arthralgia

B

due to dampness

痹而不仁［bì ér bù rén］impediment characterized by numbness of muscles

砭扁变便辨 BIAN

砭 biān

砭［biān］*Bian*-stone ~ , 以石刺病也。*Bian is* a stone used to puncture for treating disorders.

砭石［biān shí］*Bian*-stone, healing stone 治以 ~ treating with a stone needle/针法起源于古代的 ~ 。Acupuncture developed from the ancient *Bian*-stone.

砭针［biān zhēn］stone needle 采用 ~ 治疗 treating diseases with stone needles

扁 biǎn

扁平胸［biǎn píng xiōng］flat chest

变 biàn

变味［biàn wèi］going bad 肉 ~ 了。The meat has gone bad.

变证［biàn zhèng］deteriorated pattern

便 biàn

便时闭口［biàn shí bì kǒu］keeping mouth close in bowel movement ~ , 则可避免污秽气体进入口内。Keeping mouth close in bowel movement could prevent dirty gas from entering the mouth.

便数［biàn shuò］frequent bowel movements ~ 憎风 frequent bowel movements with aversion to wind

便溲［biàn sōu］excreting feces and urine ~ 不时 frequent excreting feces and urine

便血［biàn xiě］having blood in one's feces

辨 biàn

辨列星辰［biàn liè xīng chén］identifying the change of the stars 通过 ~ 调整作息, 以达养生目的。Health preservation is achieved by identifying the stars and adjusting work and rest.

辨体施食［biàn tǐ shī shí］having diet based on a person's body constitution

辨证论治［biàn zhèng lùn zhì］pattern differentiation and treatment

辨证择食［biàn zhèng zé shí］choosing food based on pattern differentiation

辨证施养［biàn zhèng shī yǎng］health preservation based on pattern differentiation

标表 BIAO

标 biāo

标本［biāo běn］superficiality and origin; symptoms and root cause ~ 兼治。Relieve the primary and secondary symptoms at the same time.

表 biǎo

表寒里热［biǎo hán lǐ rè］exterior cold and interior heat

表里［biǎo lǐ］exterior and interior ~ 双解 releasing both the exterior and in-

B

terior conditions/ ~ 同病 disease with the exterior and interior involved

表里传 [biǎo lǐ chuán] transmission from the exterior to the interior

表里俱寒 [biǎo lǐ jù hán] cold in both the exterior and interior

表里俱热 [biǎo lǐ jù rè] heat in both the exterior and interior

表里配穴 [biǎo lǐ pèi xué] combination of the exterior-interior related meridian acupoints 治疗本脏本腑有关疾病时宜采用 ~ 。 Acupoints of the exterior and interior related meridians are selected in treatment for diseases involving the same *zang-fu* organs.

表皮 [biǎo pí] outer skin

表气不固 [biǎo qì bù gù] defensive qi weakness ~ ，邪气入里化热。 When the defensive qi is weak, pathogenic factors would invade the interior and transform into heat.

表情 [biǎo qíng] expression 自信的 ~ a look of confidence

表热里寒 [biǎo rè lǐ hán] exterior heat and interior cold

表实里虚 [biǎo shí lǐ xū] exterior excess and interior deficiency

表邪入里 [biǎo xié rù lǐ] invasion of the interior by external pathogenic factors

表虚里实 [biǎo xū lǐ shí] exterior deficieny and interior excess

表证 [biǎo zhèng] exterior pattern

别 BIE

别 bié

别络 [bié luò] divergent collateral 十五 ~ fifteen divergent collaterals

别穴 [bié xué] extraordinary acupoint

冰屏饼禀并病 BING

冰 bīng

冰棍 [bīng gùn] popsicle

冰上运动 [bīng shàng yùn dòng] ice-sports

冰水 [bīng shuǐ] icy water ~ 不能寒 failure to be cooled by icy water

屏 bǐng

屏气 [bǐng qì] holding breath

屏息 [bǐng xī] holding breath

饼 bǐng

饼剂 [bǐng jì] medicated cake ~ 收载在我国现存最早的医方书《五十二病方》中。 Medicated cake was first recorded in the ancient medical book *Formulas for Fifty-two Diseases.*

禀 bǐng

禀赋 [bǐng fù] born gifts ~ 不足 poor born gifts

禀性 [bǐng xìng] natural disposition

并 bìng

并病 [bìng bìng] overlapping of disease

并发症 [bìng fā zhèng] complication 我弟弟手术后出现了 ~ 。 My brother developed complications after the surgery.

并月 [bìng yuè] bimonthly menstruation

B

病 bìng

病案[bìng àn] medical record

病痹 [bìng bì] suffering from impediment

病变[bìng biàn] pathological changes ~于色 pathological changes reflected on the complexion

病程[bìng chéng] course of disease ~长 long disease course

病处[bìng chù] diseased site

病从口入[bìng cóng kǒu rù] disease entering through the mouth 预防~, 不吃生冷食物。 Avoid eating anything raw or cold to prevent illness entering through the mouth.

病笃[bìng dǔ] critically ill

病而不得卧 [bìng ér bù dé wò] difficulty to lie on bed in illness

病而形肉脱 [bìng ér xíng ròu tuō] emaciation due to illness

病发而不足[bìng fā ér bù zú] disease caused by insufficiency of healthy qi ~,先治其标,后治其本。 If a disease is induced by deficiency of healthy qi, treat symptoms first and root cause second.

病发而有余 [bìng fā ér yǒu yú] a disease with excessive pathogenic factors ~,先治其本,后治其标。 If a disease is induced by excessive pathogenic factors, treat the root cause first and symptoms second.

病各有形 [bìng gè yǒu xíng] disease manifested differently

病根 [bìng gēn] disease cause; old complaint 他的~在于暴饮暴食。 His problem stems from crapulence. / 这是从小落下的~。 This is his childhood complaint.

病故[bìng gù] dying of illness

病号 [bìng hào] sick person ~饭 patient's diet

病后防复[bìng hòu fáng fù] preventing relapse after recovery

病机 [bìng jī] mechanism of disease, pathogenesis

病急乱投医 [bìng jí luàn tóu yī] Desperate people will try anything.

病假 [bìng jià] sick leave 请一周~。 Ask for one week's sick leave.

病间[bìng jiàn] mild disease

病进[bìng jìn] progress of disease ~而色危 progress of disease with unfavorable complexion

病久[bìng jiǔ] prolonged illness ~则传化。 If a disease lingers for a long time, it tends to deteriorate.

病来如山倒 [bìng lái rú shān dǎo] Diseases come like an avalanche. ~, 病去如抽丝。 Diseases come like an avalanche, but it takes time for them to go away.

病脉[bìng mài] abnormal pulse 知~而决生死。 The outcome of a disease is predicted from the abnormal pulse conditions.

病起[bìng qǐ] occurrence of disease ~疾风,至如砺砺。 A disease comes

like strong wind, while its attack is like roaring of thunder.

病气［bìng qì］pathogenic factors ~ 有余 excessive pathogenic factors

病情［bìng qíng］patient's condition ~ 恶化 exacerbation of the disease/他父亲的 ~ 有所好转。His father is on the mend.

病区［bìng qū］sick ward 她住在第五 ~。She stays in Sick Ward 5.

病容［bìng róng］sickly appearance 面带 ~ with a sickly look on the face

病入膏肓［bìng rù gāo huāng］disease beyond cure

病色［bìng sè］sickly complexion 察病机，视 ~，诊病脉。Determine pathogenesis, observe the sickly complexion and examine the abnormal pulse.

病深［bìng shēn］severity of disease

病生于内［bìng shēng yú nèi］disease located inside the body

病生于头［bìng shēng yú tóu］disease located inside the head

病生于阳［bìng shēng yú yáng］disease in the external part of the body

病史［bìng shǐ］medical history

病势［bìng shì］progress of disease

病痛［bìng tòng］sickness, illness, ailment 减轻 ~ alleviating the ailment

病危［bìng wēi］dangerously ill ~ 通知 critical condition notice to the patient's family

病因［bìng yīn］cause of disease ~ 不明。The cause of the disease is unknown.

病愈［bìng yù］recovery

病状［bìng zhuàng］symptom

拨玻菠剥薄髆 BO

拨 bō

拨络法［bō luò fǎ］collateral-poking ~ 是一种按摩手法。Collateral-poking is a kind of massage manipulation.

玻 bō

玻璃罐［bō li guàn］glass jar

菠 bō

菠菜［bō cài］spinach

菠萝［bō luó］pineapple ~ 汁 pineapple juice

剥 bō

剥苔［bō tāi］peeled fur 温病伤胃津，可见 ~。A peeled fur is seen in a warm-pathogen disease which impairs stomach fluid.

薄 bó

薄名利［bó míng lì］indifferent to fame and prosperity

髆 bó

髆［bó］arm; upper arm

哺补不布 BU

哺 bǔ

哺乳［bǔ rǔ］breast-feed ~ 期 breast-feed period, suckling stage

补 bǔ

补剂［bǔ jì］tonifying formula 虚证宜用 ~。Tonifying formulas are usually

B

employed to deal with deficiency patterns.

补精[bǔ jīng] supplementing essence ~ 益气 supplementing essence and reinforcing qi/ ~ 益气, 健脑益髓。 Supplement essence and reinforce qi to invigorate the brain.

补品[bǔ pǐn] tonic

补气[bǔ qì] reinforcing qi ~ 安神 reinforcing qi to calm the mind/ ~ 健脾 reinforcing qi and invigorating the spleen/ ~ 药 qi-reinforcing medicinals/ ~ 壮阳 reinforcing qi to invigorate yang

补弱[bǔ ruò] tonifying ~ 全真 tonifying and preserving healthy qi

补肾固发[bǔ shèn gù fà] tonifying the kidney to secure hair

补肾固精[bǔ shèn gù jīng] tonifying the kidney to secure essence ~ 药 herbal medicinals for tonifying the kidney to secure essence

补泻[bǔ xiè] reinforcing and reducing 针刺 ~ reinforcing and reducing manipulations in acupuncture/ ~ 兼施 with reinforcing and reducing methods

补虚[bǔ xū] tonifying in a deficiency condition ~ 泻实 tonifying in a deficiency condition and relieving excess/ ~ 固表 tonifying in a deficiency condition to strengthen the superficial resistance

补虚不留瘀[bǔ xū bù liú yū] tonifying in a deficiency concition without retaining blood stasis 治产后恶露不绝, 应当遵循 ~ 的原则。 The principle of tonifying in a deficiency condition without retaining blood stasis must be followed in treatment for postpartum lochiorrhea.

补血滋阴[bǔ xuè zī yīn] enriching blood and replenishing yin 熟地黄性温, 具有 ~ 的功效。 Shudihuang (Prepared Rehmannia Root), warm in property, has the potency of enriching blood and replenishing yin.

补益气血[bǔ yì qì xuè] reinforcing qi and enriching blood ~ 法可用于治疗气血两虚证。 Reinforcing qi and enriching blood are used for deficiency of both qi and blood.

补阴生津[bǔ yīn shēng jīn] replenishing yin to generate body fluids ~ 法可用于治疗阴液亏虚证。 Replenishing yin to generate body fluids is a therapy for deficiency of yin fluid.

补中益气[bǔ zhōng yì qì] strengthening the middle-energizer to reinforce qi ~ , 健脾止泻 reinforcing the qi of the middle-energizer to strengthen the spleen and stop diarrhea/ ~ , 升提固脱 reinforcing the qi of the middle-energizer to lift organs and prevent prolapse/ ~ 药 herbal medicinals for reinforcing the qi of the middle-energizer.

不 bù

不饱和脂肪[bù bǎo hé zhī fáng]

B

unsaturated fat

不得前后[bù dé qián hòu] difficult to excrete feces and urine

不得偃卧[bù dé yǎn wò] unable to lie flat

不定穴[bù dìng xué] *Ashi* acupoint

不拘时服[bù jū shí fú] taking a herbal decoction any time 煎汤代茶 ~ making a herbal decoction taken any time

不可胜数[bù kě shèng shǔ] numerous

不良[bù liáng] bad; unhealthy ~ 反应 adverse reaction, untoward effect

不寐[bù mèi] sleeplessness, insomnia 血虚 ~ insomnia due to blood deficiency/心烦 ~ sleeplessness due to vexation/热盛 ~ insomnia due to extreme heat

不内外因[bù nèi wài yīn] disease cause which is neither internal nor external

不时不食[bù shí bù shí] not eating unseasonal vegetables

不寿[bù shòu] short life span ~ 暴死 short life span and sudden death

不吮指[bù shǔn zhǐ] not sucking fingers 儿童应自幼养成 ~ 的卫生习惯。Children must have a good habit of not putting fingers in the mouth.

不通则痛[bù tōng zé tòng] pain due to stagnation of qi and blood 经脉气血运行不畅，~。Impeded flow of qi and blood in meridians brings about pain.

不痛不仁[bù tòng bù rén] numbness without pain ~ 者，病久入深。Numbness without pain indicates a chronic and incurable disease.

不图名利[bù tú míng lì] not seeking wealth or fame

不妄作劳[bù wàng zuò láo] avoiding overstrain and immoderate sexual life 法于阴阳，和于术数，食饮有节，起居有常，~。According to the theory of yin and yang and the methods of keeping fit, one should have proper diet, lead a regular life, and avoid overstrain and immoderate sexual life.

不为良相，当为良医[bù wéi liáng xiàng, dāng wéi liáng yī] Being a good physician is only second best to being a good prime minister.

不宜久煎[bù yí jiǔ jiān] herbal medicinal not to be decocted long 解表药及气味芳香之药 ~。Herbal medicinals to release the exterior or aromatic medicinals should not simmer for a long time.

不欲起晚，不欲多睡[bù yù qǐ wǎn, bù yù duō shuì] neither sleeping too late, nor sleeping too much

不欲饮食[bù yù yǐn shí] no desire to take food

不治[bù zhì] incurable ~ 之症 incurable disease/ ~ 已病治未病。Do not seek treatment only after people fall ill, but do active prevention while healthy. / ~ 已乱治未乱。Do not condition the body only when it dysfunctions, but take preventive measures before it happens.

布 bù

布托牵引［bù tuō qiān yǐn］cloth-wrapped traction

C

擦 CA

擦 cā

擦丹田［cā dān tián］rubbing *Dantian* ~ 可增强内脏功能。Rubbing *Dantian* strengthens the function of the internal organs.

擦法［cā fǎ］rubbing 大鱼际 ~ thenar rubbing/小鱼际 ~ hypothenar rubbing/掌 ~ palm rubbing

擦剂［cā jì］liniment 踝扭伤可以用 ~ 治疗。An ankle sprain can be treated with liniment.

擦脚心［cā jiǎo xīn］rubbing the sole center ~ 是民间养生习俗之一。Rubbing the sole center is a common practice to build up health.

擦面［cā miàn］rubbing the face ~ 可以调和气血。Rubbing the face can regulate qi and blood.

采彩踩菜 CAI

采 cǎi

采光［cǎi guāng］natural light 自然 ~ 对于保护视力很有好处。Natural light is beneficial to eyesight.

采制［cǎi zhì］gathering and processing ~ 草药。Gather medicinal herbs and prepare them for use.

彩 cǎi

彩色染发［cǎi sè rǎn fà］colored hair-dyeing

彩陶［cǎi táo］painted pottery ~ 文化 painted pottery culture

踩 cǎi

踩法［cǎi fǎ］gentle stepping ~ 是一种按摩方法。Gentle stepping is a kind of massage.

踩跷法［cǎi qiāo fǎ］gentle stepping ~ 能理筋整复, 缓急止痛, 松解粘连。The gentle stepping method is employed to relax muscles and tendons and relieve spasm, pain and adhesion.

菜 cài

菜花［cài huā］cauliflower

菜色［cài sè］famished complexion 面有 ~ looking famished

餐蚕 CAN

餐 cān

餐巾纸[cān jīn zhǐ] napkin paper

蚕 cán

蚕砂枕[cán shā zhěn] pillow filled with silkworm excrement ~ 有祛风燥湿,舒筋活络之效。A pillow filled with silkworm feces works to dissipate wind-dampness, relax tendons and remove obstruction from meridians. / ~ 用以祛风清热泻火。Pillows filled with silkworm excrement are good for expelling wind and heat.

仓苍藏 CANG

仓 cāng

仓廪[cāng lǐn] granary ~ 不藏 failure of the granary to store up/ ~ 之官 barn official, which refers to the spleen and stomach

苍 cāng

苍龙摆尾法[cāng lóng bǎi wěi fǎ] green dragon shaking tail method
苍天[cāng tiān] Heaven; blue sky ~ 不容。Heaven forbid.

藏 cáng

藏统失司[cáng tǒng shī sī] failure of the liver to store blood and that of the spleen to control blood ~ 会引起月经过多,或经期超前。Menorrhagia or advanced menstrual cycle is caused by failure of the liver to store blood and that of the spleen to control blood.

藏于精者,春不病温[cáng yú jīng zhě, chūn bù bìng wēn] vital essence preserved in winter, no occurrence of warm-pathogen disease in spring

操糙草 CAO

操 cāo

操劳[cāo láo] working hard ~ 过度 overworking oneself too much/你不用为孩子们 ~。You needn't worry about your children.
操心[cāo xīn] worrying, being concerned about

糙 cāo

糙皮病[cāo pí bìng] pellagra
糙苔[cāo tāi] coarse fur, rough coating

草 cǎo

草药[cǎo yào] herbal medicinal, materia medica ~ 店 herbal store/敷以 ~ applying herbal medicinals to a lesion

侧 CE

侧 cè

侧擦法[cè cā fǎ] lateral rubbing
侧卧[cè wò] lying on one's side

插茶察 CHA

插 chā

插花[chā huā] arranging flowers ~ 艺术 art of flower arrangement

茶 chá

茶[chá] tea 品 ~ tasting tea/养生 ~ tea

for good health/ ~为万病之药。Tea is a panacea./佛教养生与饮~有很深的渊源。Buddhist health preservation is closely related to tea drinking.

茶道[chá dào] tea ceremony, teaism ~大师 tea ceremony master/ ~文化 tea ceremony culture/ ~养生 health preservation with teaism

茶馆[chá guǎn] tea house 老舍~ Laoshe Tea House

茶剂[chá jì] medicated tea

茶具[chá jù] tea set ~鉴赏 tea set appreciation/挑选 ~ tea set selection

茶卤[chá lǔ] strong tea

茶食[chá shí] cakes and sweetmeats

茶汤[chá tāng] gruel of millet flour and sugar

茶文化[chá wén huà] tea culture 中国~历史悠久。Chinese tea culture has a long history.

茶叶枕[chá yè zhěn] pillow filled with used tea ~可以清肝降火。A pillow filled with used tea works to clear liver-fire.

茶艺[chá yì] tea ceremony ~表演 performing tea ceremony/ ~萌芽于唐代。The tea ceremony began in the Tang Dynasty (618-907).

茶友[chá yǒu] friends at a tea house ~会 tea club

茶醉[chá zuì] tea intoxication 饮茶应注意避免 ~。Do not drink too much tea to avoid tea intoxication.

察 chá

察色按脉[chá sè àn mài] observing the complexion and taking pulse

柴 CHAI
柴 chái

柴米油盐[chái mǐ yóu yán] daily necessities

禅缠产颤 CHAN
禅 chán

禅茶[chán chá] Zen tea ~就有助于平衡人们的心态。Zen tea helps balance mentality.

禅定[chán dìng] meditation with stoppage of thinking

缠 chán

缠喉风[chán hóu fēng] acute laryngeal infection ~多由脏腑炽热，邪毒内侵，风痰上涌所致。Acute laryngeal infection is mostly caused by heat retained in the *zang-fu* organs, invasion of the interior by pathogenic factors and upward attack by wind and phlegm.

缠腰火丹[chán yāo huǒ dān] herps zoster

产 chǎn

产妇[chǎn fù] woman in labor, puerpera

产门[chǎn mén] vaginal orifice

颤 chàn

颤动舌[chàn dòng shé] trembling

tongue 肝风内动可见 ~。Trembling tongue can be seen in patients with stirring of liver-wind.

长肠常敞畅 CHANG

长 cháng

长脉[cháng mài] long pulse ~有余,气逆火盛。Long pulse indicates adverse flow of qi and intense fire.

长蛇灸[cháng shé jiǔ] "long-snake" moxibustion

长生久视[cháng shēng jiǔ shì] long life with sharp eyes 癖邪不至, ~。Pathogenic factors do not attack the body, thereby long life is ensured.

长寿[cháng shòu] long life ~饮食食谱 macrobiotic diet/ ~之道 the way to achieve longevity

长夏[cháng xià] late summer ~多湿。Dampness dominates the late summer.

长针[cháng zhēn] long needle ~深刺。A long needle is applicable to deep insertion.

肠 cháng

肠风[cháng fēng] bloody feces due to external contraction

肠结[cháng jié] impeded flow of qi and blood in intestines

肠辟[cháng pì] dysentery; hemafacia

肠痈[cháng yōng] intestinal abscess; acute appendicitis

肠燥津亏[cháng zào jīn kuī] intestinal dryness and fluid depletion

常 cháng

常处静室[cháng chǔ jìng shì] frequently staying in a quiet room ~, 多听美言。Frequently stay in a quiet room and listen to good words.

常毒治病,十去其七[cháng dú zhì bìng, shí qù qí qī] If medicinals with slightly drastic action are used in treatment for diseases, they should be discontinued when seven-tenths of the pathogen is eliminated.

常服[cháng fú] everyday clothes 居家 ~ daily wear

常规疗法[cháng guī liáo fǎ] routine medical treatment

常见病[cháng jiàn bìng] common disease

常脉[cháng mài] normal pulse; normal pulse in four seasons

常人[cháng rén] ordinary person

常色[cháng sè] normal and healthy complexion

常温[cháng wēn] normal temperature

常欲小劳[cháng yù xiǎo láo] doing a little physical labor 养生 ~, 但莫大疲及强所不能堪耳。To keep fit it is necessary to do a little physical labor to the extent that one can tolerate.

敞 chǎng

敞亮[chǎng liàng] light and spacious ~的厨房 light and spacious kitchen

畅 chàng

畅饮[chàng yǐn] drinking one's fill, drinking one's content

超朝潮炒 CHAO

超 chāo

超逸［chāo yì］free and natural

超自然［chāo zì rán］supernatural ~现象 the supernatural

朝 cháo

朝向［cháo xiàng］orientation

朝阳［cháo yáng］having a southern exposure 他的书房 ~。His study faces south.

潮 cháo

潮气［cháo qì］humidity 昨天 ~很大。It was clammy yesterday.

潮热［cháo rè］tidal fever 日晡 ~ tidal fever in late afternoon/湿热 ~ tidal fever due to dampness-heat/阴虚 ~ tidal fever due to yin deficiency

潮湿［cháo shī］dampness 天气 ~ damp climate

炒 chǎo

炒［chǎo］dry-frying ~黄 dry-frying to yellow/ ~焦 dry-frying to brown/ ~炭 carbonized

炒三仙［chǎo sān xiān］dry-fried hawthorn, medicated leaven and malt

炒素［chǎo sù］stir-fried assorted vegetables

抻臣辰沉陈晨 CHEN

抻 chēn

抻筋拔骨［chēn jīn bá gǔ］stretching the tendons and bones ~ ,疏通经络。Stretch the tendons and bones to dredge meridians.

臣 chén

臣药［chén yào］deputy medicinal 桂枝是麻黄汤中的 ~。*Guizhi* (Cinnamon Branch) is the deputy medicinal in the *Mahuang* Decoction.

辰 chén

辰砂［chén shā］cinnabar

沉 chén

沉肩垂肘［chén jiān chuí zhǒu］relaxing shoulders and dropping elbows ~ 是太极拳的练习要领。Relaxing shoulders and dropping elbows are the key to practice tai chi chuan.

沉疴［chén kē］serious chronic disease

沉脉［chén mài］deep pulse ~主里证。Deep pulse indicates an interior pattern.

沉闷［chén mèn］oppressive, depressed 天气 ~ depressing weather/心情 ~ depressed feeling

沉香［chén xiāng］(*Chenxiang* Eaglewood) 国产 ~ Chinese eaglewood/ ~有行气止痛的功效。Eaglewood has the action of moving qi and killing pain.

陈 chén

陈醋［chén cù］mature vinegar

陈酒［chén jiǔ］mellow rice wine

陈米［chén mǐ］rice stocked for many years

陈年［chén nián］of long standing ~老

C

酒 old vintage rice wine

晨 chén

晨昏怡养 [chén hūn yí yǎng] enjoying relaxation at dawn and dusk

晨起食粥 [chén qǐ shí zhōu] congee taken in the morning ～ 极易吸收 Congee taken in the morning is good for absorption.

晨泄 [chén xiè] daybreak diarrhea 脾肾阳虚 ～。Daybreak diarrhea is due to yang deficiency of the spleen and kidney.

晨兴 [chén xīng] getting up in the early morning ～理荒秽,带月荷锄归。Get up early in the morning to pull up weeds, and go home with the pickaxe on shoulder in moonlight. / ～饮食未入口,不宜烟草。Cigarette smoking should be banned in the early morning before breakfast.

成乘澄 CHENG

成 chéng

成方 [chéng fāng] set formula ～加减 modification of a set formula

成年人 [chéng nián rén] adult

成药 [chéng yào] ready-made medicinal; patent drug 中 ～ Chinese ready-made medicianls/颗粒剂是中 ～ 的一种剂型 Granules are a form of Chinese ready-made medicinals.

乘 chéng

乘凉 [chéng liáng] enjoying the cool air

澄 chéng

澄神 [chéng shén] getting rid of distraction ～ 静 虑 getting rid of distraction and keeping a peaceful mind

吃眵迟持尺齿豉赤瘛 CHI

吃 chī

吃素 [chī sù] living on a vegetarian diet 她 ～,从来不沾荤腥。She is a vegetarian and never touches animal food.

吃斋 [chī zhāi] being a vegetarian for religious reasons

眵 chī

眵泪 [chī lèi] eye secretion and tears

迟 chí

迟脉 [chí mài] slow pulse

持 chí

持重 [chí zhòng] bearing heavy load ～ 远行 long journey with heavy load

尺 chǐ

尺肤 [chǐ fū] skin from the elbow to the wrist ～ 上 不 至 关 为 阴 绝。Yin exhaustion pulse is a condition in which the pulse is only perceptible at the *chi* portion and inperceptible at the *cun* and *guan* portions.

齿 chǐ

齿更 [chǐ gēng] dental transition 女子七岁,肾气盛, ～ 发长。Permanent teeth grow to replace the milk teeth with more hair in girls at the age of seven owing to abundant kidney-qi.

齿痕舌 [chǐ hén shé] scalloped (tooth-marked) tongue 脾虚水湿不化, 多见 ~ 。 Scalloped tongue is usually seen in patients with deficiency in the spleen and retained dampness.

齿衄 [chǐ nǜ] gum bleeding

齿宜常叩 [chǐ yí cháng kòu] clenching teeth frequently ~ 可防牙齿过早脱落。 Clenching teeth frequently prevents early loss of teeth.

豉 chǐ

豉饼灸 [chǐ bǐng jiǔ] fermented soybean-cake moxibustion

赤 chì

赤白带下 [chì bái dài xià] multicolored leukorrhagia 湿热下注, ~ pouring of dampness-heat and multicolored leukorrhagia

赤白肉际 [chì bái ròu jì] dorsal-ventral boundry of the hand 鱼际穴位于手内侧 ~ 处。 Yuji (LU 10) is located at the dorso-ventral boundary of the hand.

赤龙搅海 [chì lóng jiǎo hǎi] moving the tongue in the mouth

赤龙搅天池 [chì lóng jiǎo tiān chí] moving the tongue in the mouth ~ 是咽唾养生的重要方法。 Moving the tongue in the mouth is an important way for health preservation with saliva.

赤脉传睛 [chì mài chuán jīng] angular conjunctivitis

赤游丹 [chì yóu dān] wandering erysipelas

瘛 chì

瘛疭 [chì zòng] clonic convulsion

充冲虫重 CHONG

充 chōng

充血 [chōng xuè] congestion

冲 chōng

冲服 [chōng fú] taken with the strained decoction ~ 剂 soluable granules／散剂可以 ~ 。 Powder can be taken with the strained decoction.

冲剂 [chōng jì] dissolved medicine

冲脉 [chōng mài] Thoroughfare Vessel ~ 为血海 The Thoroughfare Vessel is the reservoir of blood. ／ ~ 起于胞中。 The Thoroughfare Vessel originates from the uterus.

冲任不固 [chōng rèn bù gù] insecurity of the Thoroughfare Vessel and Conception Vessel ~ 是妇人不孕、崩漏, 及孕妇胎动不安的常见病机。 Female infertility, abnormal uterine bleeding and threatened abortion are usually caused by insecurity of the Thoroughfare Vessel and Conception Vessel.

冲任失调 [chōng rèn shī tiáo] disharmony between the Thoroughfare Vessel and Conception Vessel ~ 会影响女性月经孕产和男性性活动。 Disharmony between the Thoroughfare Vessel and Conception Vessel has negative effect on female menstruation and pregnancy, and male sexuality.

虫 chóng

虫积[chóng jī] parasitic malnutrition

重 chóng

重方[chóng fāng] alternate formula

重感[chóng gǎn] being attacked again ~ 于 邪, 则 病 危 矣。 Repeat contracting pathogenic factors may make the condition worse.

重舌[chóng shé] sublingual swelling

重阳 [chóng yáng] Double Ninth Festival

重阳之人[chóng yáng zhī rén] person with excessive yang

抽 CHOU

抽 chōu

抽筋 [chōu jīn] cramp ~ 痧 eruptive pain with spasm of legs/腿 ~ cramp in the legs

抽气罐[chōu qì guàn] sucking cup

出除处杵触怵 CHU

出 chū

出汗[chū hàn] sweating

出入废则神机化灭[chū rù fèi zé shén jī huà miè] Stop of breath causes end of life.

出血[chū xuè] bleeding, hemorrhage

出针[chū zhēn] needle withdrawal ~ 法 needle withdrawal method

除 chú

除烦[chú fán] relieving restlessness ~

定惊 relieving restlessness to arrest convulsion/竹 叶 可 以 ~。 Zhuye (Bamboo Leaf) acts to relieve restlessness.

除寒湿[chú hán shī] removing cold-dampness 补 肝 肾, ~, 止 痹 痛 tonifying the liver and kidney, eliminating cold-dampness to relieve numbness and pain

除中 [chú zhōng] sudden spurt of appetite before collapse

处 chǔ

处方 [chǔ fāng] prescription ~ 加减 prescription with modification of ingredients/开 ~ making a prescription

处暑[chǔ shǔ] End of Heat

杵 chǔ

杵状指[chǔ zhuàng zhǐ] clubbed finger

触 chù

触电感 [chù diàn gǎn] electrical sensation 进针后, 时有 ~。 An electrical sensation is sometimes experienced when a needle is inserted.

触法[chù fǎ] digital palpation

怵 chù

怵惕[chù tì] fear ~ 思虑 constant fear and anxiety

揣 CHUAI

揣 chuǎi

揣法 [chuǎi fǎ] identifying acupoint location with massage

川穿传喘 CHUAN

川 chuān

川剧脸谱［chuān jù liǎn pǔ］Sichuan Opera ~ 脸谱 type of facial make-up in Sichuan Opera/欣赏 ~ ,让人身心愉悦。It makes your mood cheerful when you enjoy the types of facial make-up of Sichuan Opera.

穿 chuān

穿堂风［chuān táng fēng］draught 睡眠时,应避免 ~ 。Avoid draught when one is asleep.

传 chuán

传变［chuán biàn］transmission and change 卫气营血 ~ transmission of pathogenic factors from the defensive level to the qi, nutritive and blood levels

传承人［chuán chéng rén］successor 保护 ~ 代表性学术思想和经验。Preserve the intellecural and clinical traditions embodied in the representative successors.

传化［chuán huà］conveying and transforming

传经［chuán jīng］meridian transmission 病有 ~ 和不 ~ 之分。Some diseases may pass on from one meridian to another, but some may not.

传于后世［chuán yú hòu shì］passing on to the later generations

喘 chuǎn

喘不得卧［chuǎn bù dé wò］inability to lie down because of panting

喘促［chuǎn cù］panting

喘家［chuǎn jiā］patient susceptible to panting

喘咳［chuǎn ké］panting with coughing ~ 不得卧 unable to lie down owing to panting with coughing

喘鸣［chuǎn míng］wheezing panting

疮床 CHUANG

疮 chuāng

疮家［chuāng jiā］patient susceptible to developing sores

疮疡［chuāng yáng］pyogenic skin infection

床 chuáng

床必宽大［chuáng bì kuān dà］better to have a big-sized bed ~ ,则盛夏之气不逼。A big-sized bed helps keep away summer-heat.

垂捶 CHUI

垂 chuí

垂钓［chuí diào］fishing ~ 爱好者 fishing enthusiasts/ ~ 养生 health preservation with fishing/ ~ 是一种非常令人放松的活动。Fishing makes you relax all over.

垂肘［chuí zhǒu］dropping the elbows

捶 chuí

捶背［chuí bèi］pounding the back ~ 可舒筋活血。Pounding the back relaxes muscles and tendons to promote blood circulation.

捶法[chuí fǎ] tapping rhythmically with loose fists

捶击肩背[chuí jī jiān bèi] tapping the shoulders and back ~宜空拳。Tap the shoulders and back with loose fists.

春唇纯 CHUN

春 chūn

春分[chūn fēn] Spring Equinox ~昼夜同长。On Spring Equinox, the day is as long as the night. / ~是24个节气中的第4个节气。Spring Equinox is the 4th of the 24 solar terms.

春风[chūn fēng] spring breeze ~得意 being flushed with success/ ~拂面。Spring breeze caresses the cheeks. / ~化雨 life-giving spring breeze and rain; salutary influence of education/ ~满面 beaming with satisfaction/你看上去真是 ~ 满面! You look absolutely radiant!

春光[chūn guāng] sights and sounds in spring

春季养生[chūn jì yǎng shēng] health preservation in springtime ~应注重对肝脏的保养。It is the focus to take good care of the liver for health preservation in springtime.

春节[chūn jié] Spring Festival

春困秋乏[chūn kùn qiū fá] feeling sleepy in spring and tired in autumn 缓解 ~需要保持充足的睡眠时间和合理的体育运动。It is important to have enough sleep and rational exercises to relieve sleepiness in spring and tired feeling in autumn.

春气在经脉[chūn qì zài jīng mài] abundant qi and blood gathering in meridians in spring

春生[chūn shēng] revitalization in spring

春温[chūn wēn] warm-pathogen disease occurring in spring

春捂秋冻[chūn wǔ qiū dòng] not to change one's clothes too quickly with change of weather in early spring and autumn

春夏养阳[chūn xià yǎng yáng] nourishing yang in spring and summer ~, 秋冬养阴。Nourish yang in spring and summer and replenish yin in autumn and winter. / "冬吃萝卜夏吃姜"正是" ~ ,秋冬养阴"的体现。"Eating turnip in winter and ginger in summer" is an approach to "nourish yang in spring and summer and to replenish yin in autumn and winter".

春弦[chūn xián] wiry pulse appearing in spring 平人脉有 ~,是因阳气上升。Healthy people usually have wiry pulse in spring because of the ascent of yang-qi.

春意[chūn yì] spring in the air ~盎然。Spring is in the air. / ~阑珊 spring being on the wane

春应中规[chūn yìng zhòng guī] smooth

pulse appearing in spring

春雨贵如油［chūn yǔ guì rú yóu］spring rain being as precious as oil

春装［chūn zhuāng］spring clothes

唇 chún

唇厚人中长［chún hòu rén zhōng cháng］thick lips with long philtrum

唇裂［chún liè］harelip

唇针［chún zhēn］labial acupuncture

唇紫［chún zǐ］cyanotic lips

纯 chún

纯净［chún jìng］pure ～的空气 pure air/～灵魂 cleansing the soul/～水 purified water/～心灵 cleansing the mind

纯阳之体［chún yáng zhī tǐ］pure yang constitution 小儿为～。Infants often have pure yang constitution.

纯育［chún yù］pure breeding

瓷磁刺 CI

瓷 cí

瓷［cí］porcelain 青花～blue and white porcelain/中国是青花～的故乡。China is the hometown of blue and white porcelain.

磁 cí

磁疗仪［cí liáo yí］magneto-therapeutic device

磁穴疗法［cí xué liáo fǎ］magneto-acupuncture therapy

磁石枕［cí shí zhěn］pillow filled with magnet powder ～能明目益睛。A pillow filled with magnet powder is good for eyes.

刺 cì

刺法［cì fǎ］method of puncture 浅～shallow puncture/深～deep puncture/透～penetrable puncture/～灸法学 acupuncture and moxibustion techniques

刺禁［cì jìn］contraindication of needling 针灸医生都应当明白～。Acpuncturists must know the contraindications of needling.

刺灸法［cì jiǔ fǎ］acupuncture and moxibustion

刺络［cì luò］bloodletting puncture ～拔罐法 bloodletting puncture with cupping/实践证明，～拔罐改善了微循环障碍。Clinical practice shows that the bloodletting puncture and cupping could ameliorate the disturbance in microcirculation.

刺手［cì shǒu］needle-holding hand

刺痛［cì tòng］pricking pain

刺虚［cì xū］acupuncture applied to a patient with the deficiency pattern ～者须补其实。When acupuncture is applied to a patient with the deficiency pattern, the reinforcing method is always adopted.

刺血疗法［cì xuè liáo fǎ］meridian pricking with cupping 有实邪壅滞，采用～。Meridian pricking with cupping is employed when there are excessive pathogenic factors.

聪从丛 CONG

聪 cōng

聪耳[cōng ěr] improving hearing

从 cóng

从化[cóng huà] constitutionally influenced transformation

从治[cóng zhì] coacting treatment ~ 也是治病求本。Coacting treatment is also an approach to seek the root cause of a disease.

丛 cóng

丛刺[cóng cì] cluster needling

丛针[cóng zhēn] group needle

腠 COU

腠 còu

腠理[còu lǐ] striated layer ~ 闭郁 closed striated layer/ ~ 闭塞 blocked muscular interstices/ ~ 疏松 loose striated layer/ ~ 致密 compact muscular interstices/ ~ 失固,易受外邪。Insecurity of the striated layer results in easy attack by external pathogenic factors.

促醋蹴猝 CU

促 cù

促脉[cù mài] irregular rapid pulse 心阳闭阻,见 ~。Irregular rapid pulse is found in obstruction of heart-yang.

醋 cù

醋炙[cù zhì] processed with vinegar

蹴 cù

蹴鞠[cù jū] kicking a ball 中国古代的 ~ 就是世界上最早的足球运动。The earliest foolball in the world developed in ancient China, the so called "kicking a ball" at that time.

猝 cù

猝然[cù rán] suddenly ~ 暴死 sudden death

猝死[cù sǐ] sudden death

窜 CUAN

窜 cuàn

窜痛[cuàn tòng] scurrying pain

催脆焠 CUI

催 cuī

催气[cuī qì] hastening qi ~ 法 hastening qi manipulation

脆 cuì

脆脚[cuì jiǎo] swollen legs in pregnancy

焠 cuì

焠刺法[cuì cì fǎ] red-hot needling

皲存寸 CUN

皲 cūn

皲裂[cūn liè] chap 这孩子的双唇都 ~ 了。The child's lips were chapped.

存 cún

存想[cún xiǎng] mind concentration on something ~ 具有调动潜能和祛病健身的作用。Mind concentration functions to mobilize potentials and ward off diseases.

寸 cùn

寸口脉［cùn kǒu mài］wrist pulse

搓痤错 CUO

搓 cuō

搓［cuō］rubbing, scrubbing

搓背［cuō bèi］scrubbing the back ~ 能提升阳气。Scrubbing the back can ascend yang-qi.

搓柄法［cuō bǐng fǎ］handle-twisting

搓法［cuō fǎ］twisting ~ 是由摩法衍生而出的。Twisting is derived from the palm-rubbing technique.

搓滚舒筋［cuō gǔn shū jīn］twisting and rolling for tendon relaxation

搓揉头皮［cuō róu tóu pí］rubbing and kneading the scalp ~ 可缓解脱发 Baldness is relieved by rubbing and kneading the scalp.

搓针［cuō zhēn］needle twisting

痤 cuó

痤疮［cuó chuāng］acne

错 cuò

错语［cuò yǔ］disordered speech 热扰神明，~。Disordered speech results from mental activities disturbed by heat.

D

搭打大 DA

搭 dā

搭鹊桥［dā què qiáo］building the magpie bridge ~ 有沟通任督二脉之功效。Building the magpie bridge helps with communication between the Conception Vessel and Governor Vessel.

打 dǎ

打猎［dǎ liè］hunting

大 dà

大便通畅［dà biàn tōng chàng］free bowel movement ~ 是健身之要。Free bowel movement is essential for fitness. /为保证 ~ , 可选用传统保健功法，腹部按摩保健等。To maintain free bowel movement, people may do some traditional health-preserving *qigong*, abdominal massage and so on.

大补元气［dà bǔ yuán qì］reinforcing original qi ~ , 止泻固脱 reinforcing original qi to check diarrhea and rescue one from collapse

大肠［dà cháng］large intestine ~ 主传导。The large intestine is in charge of conveyance of wastes.

大肠经 [dà cháng jīng] Large Intestine Meridian

大肠咳 [dà cháng ké] feces incontinence in coughing

大肠湿热 [dà cháng shī rè] dampness-heat in the large intestine

大出血 [dà chū xuè] massive hemorrhage

大动肝火 [dà dòng gān huǒ] flying into a rage

大毒治病，十去其六 [dà dú zhì bìng, shí qù qí liù] If medicinals with drastic action are used in treatment for diseases, they should be discontinued when six-tenths of the pathogens is eliminated.

大寒 [dà hán] Great Cold

大厥 [dà jué] coma in stroke

大络 [dà luò] large collateral 十五~ fifteen large collaterals

大脉 [dà mài] large pulse ~则病近。 Large pulse indicates deterioration of a disease.

大怒则行气绝 [dà nù zé xíng qì jué] Sudden fainting is caused by fury resulting in qi exhaustion and blood rushing up to the head.

大肉 [dà ròu] pork

大实有羸状 [dà shí yǒu léi zhuàng] pseudo-deficiency manifestations seen in an extreme excess pattern ~, 至虚有盛候 pseudo-deficiency manifestations seen in an extreme excess pattern and manifestations of a pseudo-excess pattern appearing in an extreme deficiency pattern

大暑 [dà shǔ] Great Heat

大头瘟 [dà tóu wēn] infectious swollen head

大雪 [dà xuě] Great Snow

大医精诚 [dà yī jīng chéng] perfect proficiency of a great doctor

大疫 [dà yì] pandemic 孟春行秋令，则民~。 If in the first month of spring there is autumn-like weather, pandemic will prevail.

大针 [dà zhēn] big needle

大周天 [dà zhōu tiān] macro-cosmic orbit, large heavenly circuit 打通 ~ dredging the macro-cosmic orbit

呆傣代带戴 DAI

呆 dāi

呆小症 [dāi xiǎo zhèng] cretinism

呆滞 [dāi zhì] dull, lifeless 目光~with a blank look in one's eyes

傣 dǎi

傣医学 [dǎi yī xué] Dai ethnic medicine

代 dài

代脉 [dài mài] regularly intermittent pulse ~主脏气变微。 Regularly intermittent pulse suggests exhaustion of qi of the *zang*-organs.

D

带 dài

带脉［dài mài］Belt Vessel ~ 约束诸脉。The Belt Vessel controls all the meridians. / ~ 起于季肋部，横行环绕腰部一周。The Belt Vessel, originating from the hypochondrial region, runs transversely around the waist.

带下臭秽［dài xià chòu huì］foul leukorrhea 肾虚 ~ 淋漓 dribbling foul leukorrhea due to deficiency in the kidney

戴 dài

戴红布［dài hóng bù］wearing a piece of red cloth 今人 ~ 抹胸，云可养心血即是。It is said that wearing a piece of red cloth around the chest nourishes heart blood.

戴阳［dài yáng］floating of yang

丹单胆旦淡但 DAN

丹 dān

丹毒［dān dú］erysipelas

丹剂［dān jì］vermillion pill, pellet

丹痧［dān shā］scarlet fever

丹田［dān tián］the pubic region, *Dantian* ~ 呼吸法 fetal breathing / 上、中、下 ~ upper, middle and lower *Dantian* / 意守 ~ mind concentration on *Dantian*

单 dān

单方［dān fāng］simple formula ~ 药少力专。A simple formula usually consists of a few herbal ingredients with an extraordinary effect.

单煎［dān jiān］decocted alone 人参等贵重药材在煎煮时需要 ~。Fine medicinals like ginseng should better be decocted alone.

胆 dǎn

胆经［dǎn jīng］Gallbladder Meridian

胆咳［dǎn ké］coughing up bile

胆热［dǎn rè］gallbladder-heat

胆郁痰扰证［dǎn yù tán rǎo zhèng］pattern of stagnation of gallbladder-qi and phlegm disturbance

胆主决断［dǎn zhǔ jué duàn］gallbladder controlling the capacity of making a decision

旦 dàn

旦发夕死［dàn fā xī sǐ］dying in a short time

旦慧［dàn huì］alleviating in the morning ~ 昼安 alleviating in the morning and well in the daytime

淡 dàn

淡泊［dàn bó］not interested in fame or wealth ~ 名利 indifferent to fame or wealth

淡然无为［dàn rán wú wéi］being peaceful and accomplishing nothing

淡渗利湿［dàn shèn lì shī］administering herbal medicinals milder in flavor to eliminate dampness

淡渗利水［dàn shèn lì shuǐ］administering herbal medicinals milder in flavor for diuresis ~ 消肿

administering herbal medicinals milder in flavor for diuresis to eliminate edema/茯苓 ~,健脾消肿。 *Fuling* (Indian Bread) acts to increase discharge of . urine, strengthen the spleen and eliminate edema.

但 dàn

但寒不热 [dàn hán bù rè] chills without fever

但热不寒[dàn rè bù hán] fever without chills

但欲寐[dàn yù mèi] somnolence 阴盛 阳衰之 ~ somnolence due to excessive yin and declined yang 少阴 之为病,脉微细, ~ 。 Somnolence with a thready pulse is seen in disorders of the *Shaoyin* Meridian.

当 DANG

当 dāng

当令[dāng lìng] being in season 现在 西瓜正 ~ 。 Watermelon is in season just now.

刀导捣倒倒盗道 DAO

刀 dāo

刀针[dāo zhēn] knife needle

导 dǎo

导气[dǎo qì] guiding qi ~ 下行 guiding qi downward

导药[dǎo yào] medicinals that induce bowel movement

导引 [dǎo yǐn] *Daoyin*, conduction exercise 按摩 ~ 健身法 remedial massage and *qigong* with the conduction exercise to keep fit

捣 dǎo

捣碎[dǎo suì] pounding to pieces

捣针[dǎo zhēn] repeating needle lifting and thrusting

倒 dǎo

倒法 [dǎo fǎ] pulling in opposite direction

倒 dào

倒经[dào jīng] vicarious menstruation

盗 dào

盗汗[dào hàn] night sweating

道 dào

道、术、法、势[dào, shù, fǎ, shì] morality, ruling methods, law and power

道德 [dào dé] virtue; way of health preservation 中古之世, ~ 稍衰。 In the middle ancient times the theory of health preservation declined.

道地药材 [dào dì yào cái] authenic medicinal substances

道法自然 [dào fǎ zì rán] divine law following nature 人法地,地法天,天 法道, ~ 。Man imitates earth. Earth imitates heaven. Heaven follows the divine law, and the divine law follows nature.

得 DE

得 dé

得道[dé dào] just cause ~ 多助,失道

D

寡助。A just cause enjoys abundant support while an unjust cause finds little. /非其人不教,非其真不授,是谓 ~。Do not teach these abstruse theories to anyone not eligible or unqualified to study them. This is the right way to pass on such valuable theories.

得气 [dé qì] arrival of qi ~ 反应 presence of arrival of qi/ ~ 是指针刺入腧穴后,通过某些手法使针刺部位产生特殊的感觉。Arrival of qi refers to a special sensation produced in the area after acupuncture and certain manipulations are applied.

得神 [dé shén] full of vitality ~ 者昌。Patients with vitality are prone to be cured.

得意忘象 [dé yì wàng xiàng] getting the real meaning and forgetting the image

登等 DENG

登 dēng

登高 [dēng gāo] ascending a height ~ 节 Height Ascending Festival/ ~ 望远 ascending a height to view distant places/ ~ 是重阳节很重要的活动。Ascending a height is one of the most important activities on the Double Ninth Festival.

等 děng

等分 [děng fēn] equal amount ~ 为末 powder divided into equal portions

滴地 DI

滴 dī

滴剂 [dī jì] drop 鼻炎可以用 ~ 治疗。Rhinitis is treated with drops.

滴酒法 [dī jiǔ fǎ] alcohol burning cupping

滴丸 [dī wán] dripping pill 丹参 ~ *Danshen* Dripping Pills

地 dì

地老天荒 [dì lǎo tiān huāng] till the end of the world

地势 [dì shì] topography, terrain ~ 平缓 smooth terrain/ ~ 险要 strategically important terrain that is difficult to access

地图舌 [dì tú shé] map tongue

地支 [dì zhī] Earthly Branches

癫颠碘点踮电 DIAN

癫 diān

癫病 [diān bìng] depressive psychosis; epilepsy

颠 diān

颠顶 [diān dǐng] parietal bone

碘 diǎn

碘酒 [diǎn jiǔ] iodine tincture

点 diǎn

点刺 [diǎn cì] acupoint pricking ~ 疗法 acupoint pricking therapy/ ~ 用于放血疗法。The acupoint pricking method is used for bloodletting.

点刺舌[diǎn cì shé] spotted tongue

点心[diǎn xīn] dessert, dim sum

点穴 [diǎn xué] digital acupoint pressure ~ 弹筋法 acupoint massage and tendon rebound technique

点压推拿法[diǎn yā tuī ná fǎ] digital acupoint pressing with massage ~ 也可以用于治疗脏腑疾患。Digital acupoint pressing with massage is also used to treat disorders of the *zang-fu* organs.

踮 diǎn

踮足[diǎn zú] standing on tiptoe 引颈 ~ stretching out one's neck and standing on tiptoe

电 diàn

电按摩法 [diàn àn mó fǎ] electro-massage

电灸 [diàn jiǔ] electro-moxibustion ~ 仪 electro-moxibustion apparatus/ ~ 治疗简便, 成本低廉, 毒副作用小, 易于被患者接受。Electro-moxibustion is easy to operate with low cost and minor side effect, so it is welcomed by patients.

电热针[diàn rè zhēn] electrothermic needle ~灸 electrothermic needling

电针[diàn zhēn] electro-acupuncture ~ 疗法 electro-acupuncture therapy/ ~ 麻醉 electroacupuncture anesthesia/ 探讨 ~对膝骨关节炎软骨修复的影响。Investigate the effect of electro-acupuncture on cartilage renovation in knee osteoarthritis.

吊掉 DIAO

吊 diào

吊脚楼 [diào jiǎo lóu] house propped up by wooden supports with ladders leading up

掉 diào

掉眩[diào xuàn] dizziness with shaking of the head and limbs

跌 DIE

跌 diē

跌打损伤[diē dǎ sǔn shāng] traumatic injury ~包括刀枪、跌仆、殴打、内压等。Traumatic injury includes injuries caused by sharp instruments, fall and stumble, beating up and internal pressure.

疗酊锭定 DING

疗 dīng

疗[dīng] deep-rooted boil; furuncle

酊 dīng

酊剂[dīng jì] tincture ~ 可以用来消毒。Tincture is used for disinfection.

锭 dìng

锭剂[dìng jì] lozenge ~ 的作用比汤剂慢。The action of a lozenge is milder than that of a herbal decoction.

定 dìng

定境[dìng jìng] quiet state of the mind

东冬动冻洞 DONG

东 dōng

东医[dōng yī] oriental medicine

冬 dōng

冬病夏治[dōng bìng xià zhì] preventing potentials of disease occurring in winter with treatment in summer.

冬藏[dōng cáng] storing up yang-qi in winter

冬季养生[dōng jì yǎng shēng] health preservation in winter

冬令进补[dōng lìng jìn bǔ] taking tonics in winter

冬脉在骨[dōng mài zài gǔ] pulse seated deeply in winter

冬暖夏凉[dōng nuǎn xià liáng]（of climate）warm in winter and cool in summer ~的居所有利于保养健康。A residence warm in winter and cool in summer is good for health.

冬伤于寒,春必病温[dōng shāng yú hán, chūn bì bìng wēn] Attacked by pathogenic cold in winter, one will contract a warm-pathogen disease in spring.

冬石[dōng shí] normally deep pulse seen in winter

冬温[dōng wēn] warm-pathogen disease occurring in winter ~是一种热性病。Warm-pathogen disease occurring in winter is a febrile disease.

冬宜食牛羊[dōng yí shí niú yáng] better to eat more beef and lamb in winter

冬应中权[dōng yìng zhòng quán] pulse appearing deep in winter

冬至[dōng zhì] Winter Solstice ~寓意寒冷将至。Winter Solstice refers to coming of severe cold. / ~有吃水饺、汤圆、喝羊肉汤的传统习俗。On the day of Winter Solstice the Chinese people have a custom to eat *jiao zi*, sweet dumplings or drink lamb soup.

动 dòng

动功 [dòng gōng] dynamic *qigong*, motion *qigong* 四十九式经络 ~ 49-styled meridian dynamic *qigong*

动静不失其时[dòng jìng bù shī qí shí] proper combination of the dynamic and static state

动静结合 [dòng jìng jié hé] combination of the dynamic and static state 骨折的治疗宜 ~。In treatment for fracture, it is necessary to combine the dynamic with static state. / ~指在气功和武术中,静功和动功互相配合,效果显著。In *qigong* and martial arts combination of the dynamic and static state presents good effect.

动静适宜 [dòng jìng shì yí] appropriately dynamic and static state

动静相兼功[dòng jìng xiāng jiān gōng] dynamic-static *qigong*

动静有常[dòng jìng yǒu cháng] rules of the dynamic and static state

动脉[dòng mài] stirred pulse; arterial pulsation

动随意行 [dòng suí yì xíng] body movements controlled by the mind ~是气功的基本要领。Body movement controlled by the mind is the key point in doing *qigong* exercise.

动形 [dòng xíng] body exercise

动辄汗出 [dòng zhé hàn chū] sweating on minimal exertion ~ 可见于气虚证。Sweating on minimal exertion is usually seen in the qi deficiency pattern.

动中有静 [dòng zhōng yǒu jìng] quiescence within motion

冻 dòng

冻疮 [dòng chuāng] frostbite 手足 ~ frostbite on the hand and foot

洞 dòng

洞泄 [dòng xiè] severe diarrhea

抖 DOU
抖 dǒu

抖法 [dǒu fǎ] shaking maneuver ~ 用于疏松脉络, 滑利关节。The shaking maneuver is used to dredge meridians and lubricate joints.

督独毒读肚 DU
督 dū

督脉 [dū mài] Governor Vessel ~ 为阳脉之海。The Governor Vessel is the reservoir of the yang meridians.

独 dú

独立守神 [dú lì shǒu shén] keeping a sound mind

独语 [dú yǔ] soliloquy

毒 dú

毒性 [dú xìng] toxicity ~ 反应 toxic

reaction/乌头的 ~ 反应很强烈。The toxic reaction of *Wutou* (Monkshood) is very strong.

毒药 [dú yào] poison

读 dú

读书悦心 [dú shū yuè xīn] a feeling of delight accompanied by reading

肚 dù

肚兜 [dù dōu] diomand-shaped undergarment covering the abdomen and chest

肚脐 [dù qí] umbilicus, navel 神阙位于 ~ 中央。Shenque (GV 8) is sited on the center of the umbilicus.

端短断 DUAN
端 duān

端午节 [duān wǔ jié] Dragon Boat Festival

端正坐姿 [duān zhèng zuò zī] straight sitting ~ 防脊柱侧弯。Straight sitting prevents scoliosis.

短 duǎn

短刺 [duǎn cì] short thrusting of a needle

短脉 [duǎn mài] short pulse ~ 气病。Short pulse indicates qi disorder.

短缩舌 [duǎn suō shé] contracted tongue

断 duàn

断心 [duàn xīn] dismissing obsession 佛谓之曰:若断其阴, 不如 ~ 。The Buddha says: It's better to abandon wishful thinking of sex rather than cutting off the private parts.

对 DUI
对 duì
对症下药［duì zhèng xià yào］administering specific medications for an illness

顿 DUN
顿 dùn
顿服［dùn fú］taken at a draught 桂枝甘草汤需要 ~。The *Guizhi Gancao Decoction* should be taken at a draught.
顿咳［dùn ké］paroxysmal cough

多夺度 DUO
多 duō
多汗［duō hàn］profuse sweating ~ 伤阴。Profuse sweating impairs yin.
多念则智散［duō niàn zé zhì sàn］wisdom exhaustion due to too many ideas 多思则神殆，~。Worry beyond measure leads to mental weariness and illness, and too many ideas result in wisdom exhaustion.
多尿［duō niào］excessive secretion of urine, polyuria
多食［duō shí］excessive eating, polyphagia
多事则劳形［duō shì zé láo xíng］physical fatigue caused by overwork
多阴之人［duō yīn zhī rén］person with much yin
多饮［duō yǐn］excessive thirst and fluid intake, polydipsia ~ 数小便 frequent urination caused by excessive fluid intake
多欲则智昏［duō yù zé zhì hūn］being blinded by strong desire
多针浅刺［duō zhēn qiǎn cì］superficial multiple needling ~ 可治局部痒、麻木。Superficial multiple needling may treat topical itching and numbness.

夺 duó
夺精［duó jīng］essence depletion
夺气［duó qì］qi depletion
夺血［duó xuè］loss of blood ~ 者无汗 Those who suffer from loss of blood do not sweat.

度 duó
度其形之肥瘦［duó qí xíng zhī féi shòu］consideration of the patient's body build
度事上下［duó shì shàng xià］In diagnosis take into consideration of the condition of the upper and lower part of the patient's body.

E

鹅恶呃遏腭 E

鹅 é

鹅口疮[é kǒu chuāng] thrush

恶 è

恶露[è lù] lochia ～不尽 lochiorrhea/ ～不下 lochioschesis

恶脉[è mài] extremely dangerous pulse quality ～表示病情危重。Very dangerous pulse quality points to a critical case.

恶色[è sè] sickly complexion ～现,胃气枯竭,预后不良。Presence of sickly complexion refers to exhaustion of stomach-qi and poor prognosis.

恶血[è xuè] putrid blood ～不除,新血不生 no elimination of putrid blood, no production of new blood/ ～阻滞胞宫 putrid blood retained in the uterus

恶阻[è zǔ] severe morning sickness

呃 è

呃逆[è nì] hiccuping

遏 è

遏阳[è yáng] inhibited flow of yang-qi

腭 è

腭裂[è liè] cleft palate

儿耳二 ER

儿 ér

儿枕痛[ér zhěn tòng] abdominal pain after childbirth

耳 ěr

耳[ěr] ear ～廓 auricle/ ～轮 helix/ ～垂 earlobe/ ～膜 eardrum/ ～屏 tragus/ ～窍 external auditory meatus

耳聪目明[ěr cōng mù míng] having good eyes and ears 这位老人已年过七旬,仍然 ～。The old man is already over seventy, but he still has good ears and eyes.

耳目不明[ěr mù bù míng] deafness with blurred vision

耳目聪明[ěr mù cōng míng] good hearing and keen vision

耳勿极听[ěr wù jí tīng] avoiding intolerable noise ～以保护听力。Avoid intolerable noise to protect one's hearing.

耳宜常拧[ěr yí cháng níng] kneading ears often ～,且凝神去杂念,可去头旋之病。Kneading ears often may help clear distracting thoughts and take away dizziness and vertigo.

耳宜常弹[ěr yí cháng tán] flicking ears frequently ～可防治耳聋、耳鸣。

Flicking ears frequently prevents deafness and tinnitus.

耳针［ěr zhēn］ ear (auricular) acupuncture ~ 疗法 ear acupuncture therapy/ ~ 镇痛 ear acupuncture analgesia

二 èr

二便［èr biàn］ feces and urine ~ 通利 normal urination and defecation/ ~ 不利 difficulty in urination and defecation/ ~ 失禁 urine and feces incontinence

二十八脉［èr shí bā mài］ twenty-eight pulse qualities

二十八宿［èr shí bā xiù］ twenty-eight constellations

F

F

发法发 FA
发 fā

发陈［fā chén］ emergence of yang-qi 春三月，此谓 ~ 。During the three months of spring, yang-qi emerges.

发糕［fā gāo］ steamed sponge cake

发汗解表［fā hàn jiě biǎo］ inducing sweating to release the exterior ~ ，兼降逆止呕 inducing sweating to release the exterior and bringing down adverse flow of qi to stop vomiting

发酵［fā jiào］ fermenting ~ 酒 fermented wine/ ~ 茶 fermented tea

发霉［fā méi］ going mouldy ~ 的蛋糕 mouldy cake

发面［fā miàn］ leavening dough ~ 饼 leavened pancake

发胖［fā pàng］ getting on weight

发疱［fā pào］ vesiculation ~ 灸 vesiculating moxibustion/在本研究中，我们发现 ~ 灸对于已知过敏原的过敏性鼻炎患者具有较好的治疗效果。Our study finds vesiculating moxibustion is more effective in treating patients with allergic rhinitis with known allergens.

发气［fā qì］ (for a *qigong* master) emission of qi ~ 手法 qi emission maneuver

发热恶寒［fā rè wù hán］ fever and aversion to cold ~ 而疟 malaria marked by alternate fever and chill

发散［fā sàn］ dissipating ~ 表邪 dissipating superficial pathogenic factors

发酸［fā suān］ going sour 牛奶 ~ 了。The milk has gone sour.

发物［fā wù］ stimulating food 一些疾病禁止食用 ~ 。Patients with some

diseases are not allowed to have stimulating food.

发颐［fā yí］ mumps；pyogenic inflammation of the cheek

法 fǎ

法四时［fǎ sì shí］following the changes of the four seasons ~ 而治疗 medical treatment based on the changes of the four seasons

法天则地［fǎ tiān zé dì］abiding by the law of the Heaven and Earth ~ , 合以天光。Abide by the law of the Heaven and Earth and follow the movement of the celestial bodies.

法于往古［fǎ yú wǎng gǔ］following the experience of ancient practice ~ , 验于今来 Learn the ancient theory and put it into practice in current medical treatment.

法于阴阳［fǎ yú yīn yáng］following the rule of yin and yang

发 fà

发为血之余［fà wéi xuè zhī yú］hair, the surplus of blood

发宜多梳［fà yí duō shū］combing hair frequently ~ 能起到疏通头皮脉络，防止脱发的效果。Combing hair frequently is helpful for dredging meridians on the head and preventing hair loss.

发长［fà zhǎng］growth of hair

发质干枯［fà zhì gān kū］withered hair 肝肾阴虚导致的 ~ 。Yin deficiency of the liver and kidney leads to withered hair.

烦蕃凡燔反返犯饭泛 FAN

烦 fán

烦渴［fán kě］extreme thirst

烦心［fán xīn］annoying ~ 短气 annoying with shortness of breath/ ~ 胸中热 annoying with a feverish sensation in the chest/你有什么 ~ 事？What's bothering you?

蕃 fán

蕃秀［fán xiù］yang-qi developing 夏三月,此谓 ~ 。During the three months of summer, yang-qi develops.

凡 fán

凡欲眠,勿歌咏［fán yù mián, wù gē yǒng］not singing before going to bed

燔 fán

燔针法［fán zhēn fǎ］burnt needle method

反 fǎn

反复［fǎn fù］recurrence ~ 发作 repeated attack

反关脉［fǎn guān mài］pulse on the back of the wrist

反季节［fǎn jì jié］out of season ~ 蔬菜 out-of-season vegetables

反酸［fǎn suān］casting up of gastric acid

反胃［fǎn wèi］feeling queasy 病人反胃想呕吐。The patient's stomach churned and he felt sick. /我老是 ~ 。I keep regurgitating.

反治［fǎn zhì］paradoxical treatment

反佐［fǎn zuǒ］using corrigent ~是中医遣方选药的一种方法。Using corrigents is an approach to selection of herbal medicinals in traditional Chinese medicine.

返 fǎn

返老还童［fǎn lǎo huán tóng］recovering one's youthful vigor

返璞归真［fǎn pú guī zhēn］returning to nature

犯 fàn

犯贼风［fàn zéi fēng］invasion by pathogenic wind when one is in boor health ~虚邪者，阳受之。The yang meridian is attacked by pathogenic wind and other factors in a deficiency condition.

饭 fàn

饭必小咽［fàn bì xiǎo yàn］swallowing food slowly 凡养生，~，食必定量。To enjoy good health, one must swallow food slowly and have meals of fixed quantity.

饭后服［fàn hòu fú］taking after meals

饭前服［fàn qián fú］taking before meals

泛 fàn

泛舟［fàn zhōu］going boating ~湖上 going boating on a lake

方芳防房放 FANG

方 fāng

方便食品［fāng biàn shí pǐn］convenience food

方剂［fāng jì］formula

方食无饮［fāng shí wú yǐn］not taking a herbal decoction right after food intake

方士［fāng shì］diviner; alchemist

方书［fāng shū］books on Chinese formulas

方饮无食［fāng yǐn wú shí］not to take any food right after taking a herbal decoction

芳 fāng

芳香化湿［fāng xiāng huà shī］resolving dampness with aromatic herbal medicinals

芳香开窍［fāng xiāng kāi qiào］inducing resuscitation with aromatic herbal medicinals

芳香药［fāng xiāng yào］aromatic herbal medicinals ~能透表里之湿。Aromatic herbal medicinals act to eliminate internal or external dampness. / ~善走窜，祛散外邪。Since they have the dissipating action, aromatic herbal medicinals can eliminate external pathogenic factors.

防 fáng

防尘［fáng chén］being dustproof ~罩 dust cover

防风御寒［fáng fēng yù hán］keeping out wind and cold 注重 ~有助于养生。Keeping out wind and cold is good for health preservation.

防患于未然［fáng huàn yú wèi rán］nipping in the bud 只有 ~，我们才不

F

致吃亏。Only nip it in bud can we avoid losses.

防老[fáng lǎo] preparing for one's old age 养儿 ~，积谷防荒。Bring up boys to take care of their elderly parents and stockpile grains against lean years.

防暑[fáng shǔ] heat-stroke prevention ~ 降温 heat-stroke control/ ~ 措施 measures taken to prevent heat-stroke/ ~ 药 heat-stroke preventives

防治 [fáng zhì] prevention and treatment ~ 方法 method of prevention and treatment/ ~ 原则 principle for prevention and treatment/ ~ 疾病的药物主要来自植物、矿物和动物。Medicinal substances used to prevent and treat diseases come mostly from plants, minerals and animals.

防皱增颜[fáng zhòu zēng yán] wrinkle prevention to strengthen beautiful appearance

房 fáng

房劳宜节 [fáng láo yí jié] avoiding sexual overindulgence

房事[fáng shì] sexual intercourse 节制 ~ restricting sexual intercourse

房中[fáng zhōng] sexual intercourse 房中术 art of sexual intercourse

放 fàng

放松 [fàng sōng] relaxation ~ 肌肉 relaxing muscles/全身 ~ relaxing all over/逐步 ~ relaxing one part after another/ ~ 功 relaxation *qigong*

肥肺沸 FEI

肥 féi

肥人 [féi rén] obese people ~ 湿多。Obese people often have much dampness.

肥者令人内热[féi zhě lìng rén nèi rè] internal heat caused by eating too much rich food ~，甘者令人中满。Excessive greasy food causes production of internal heat and excessive sweet food causes abdominal distension.

肺 fèi

肺[fèi] lung ~ 气 lung-qi/ ~ 津 lung-fluid/ ~ 阴 lung-yin/ ~ 阳 lung-yang/ ~ 主通调水道。The lung dominates dredging the water passage.

肺病禁苦[fèi bìng jìn kǔ] bitter flavor abstained in patients with lung disease

肺藏魄 [fèi cáng pò] corporeal soul stored in the lung

肺朝百脉 [fèi cháo bǎi mài] all blood vessels leading to the lung ~，输精于皮毛。All blood vessels lead to the lung, and essence is distributed to the skin and hair.

肺合大肠 [fèi hé dà cháng] lung and large intestine in pair

肺合皮毛 [fèi hé pí máo] lung being closely related to the skin and hair

肺津亏损[fèi jīn kuī sǔn] loss of lung-fluid

肺经[fèi jīng] Lung Meridian

肺开窍于鼻[fèi kāi qiào yú bí] nose, the window of the lung

肺咳[fèi ké] cough due to lung disorder

肺苦气上逆[fèi kǔ qì shàng nì] lung often suffering from adverse rise of lung-qi ~, 急食苦以泄之。The lung often suffers from adverse rise of lung-qi, but it can be cured by immediate taking food or medicinals bitter in flavor.

肺痨[fèi láo] pulmonary tuberculosis

肺气不宣[fèi qì bù xuān] failure of lung-qi to ventilate

肺气壅滞[fèi qì yōng zhì] plugged lung-qi

肺热便秘[fèi rè biàn mì] constipation due to lung-heat

肺热炽盛证[fèi rè chì shèng zhèng] intense lung-heat pattern

肺肾气虚[fèi shèn qì xū] deficiency of lung-qi and kidney-qi

肺肾阴虚[fèi shèn yīn xū] deficiency of lung-yin and kidney-yin

肺失清肃[fèi shī qīng sù] impairment of the purifying and descending function of the lung

肺为娇脏[fèi wéi jiāo zàng] lung, the delicate *zang*-organ

肺为水之上源[fèi wèi shuǐ zhī shàng yuán] lung, the upper source of water

肺痿[fèi wěi] lung atrophy

肺痈[fèi yōng] pulmonary abscess

肺与大肠相表里[fèi yǔ dà cháng xiāng biǎo lǐ] exterior-interior relationship between the lung and large intestine

肺胀[fèi zhàng] lung distension

肺主气[fèi zhǔ qì] qi ruled by the lung

沸 fèi

沸水冲化[fèi shuǐ chōng huà] infusing with boiling water 颗粒药物应 ~ 服用。Granulated medicnals are taken after being infused in boiling water.

分焚粉 FEN

分 fēn

分刺[fēn cì] needling applied to the muscular space

分筋[fēn jīn] separating adhesive soft tissues

分肉[fēn ròu] boundary between muscles

焚 fén

焚香[fén xiāng] burning incense ~ 祭奠 burning incense and holding a memorial service/沐浴 ~ taking a bath and burning incense

粉 fěn

粉刺[fěn cì] acne ~ 常因肺经血热而成。Blood-heat in the Lung Meridian always results in acne.

丰风封锋缝 FENG

丰 fēng

丰乳[fēng rǔ] enlarging the breast

风 fēng

风关[fēng guān] wind pass

风寒[fēng hán] pathogenic wind-cold ~

F

束肺 lung fettered by wind-cold

风寒犯肺 [fēng hán fàn fèi] invasion of the lung by wind-cold

风火 [fēng huǒ] pathogenic wind-fire ~ 相煽 incitement between wind and fire

风火眼 [fēng huǒ yǎn] acute conjunctivitis, wind-fire eye, pink eye ~ 痛 painful pink eye

风家 [fēng jiā] one susceptible to wind

风热 [fēng rè] pathogenic wind-heat ~ 头痛 headache due to wind-heat

风善行而数变 [fēng shàn xíng ér shuò biàn] Wind moves swiftly and is changeable.

风胜则动 [fēng shèng zé dòng] involuntary movements induced by prevalence of wind

风湿 [fēng shī] pathogenic wind-dampness ~ 病 rheumatic disease/ ~ 性关节炎 rheumatic arthritis

风水 [fēng shuǐ] geomantic omen, feng shui ~ 宝地 a place of excellent geomantic quality/ ~ 理论 theory of geomantic omen/ ~ 先生 feng shui master, geomancer /看 ~ practicing feng shui

风水相搏 [fēng shuǐ xiāng bó] wind-water combat

风团 [fēng tuán] wheal

风为百病之长 [fēng wéi bǎi bìng zhī zhǎng] wind, the dominant factor causing various diseases ~ , 所以要注意避风保暖。 It is essential to take shelter from wind and keep warm since wind is the dominant factor causing various diseases.

风味菜 [fēng wèi cài] local delicacies

风味小吃 [fēng wèi xiǎo chī] local snacks, local delicacies

风温 [fēng wēn] wind-warm pathogen; wind-warm pathogen disease ~ 首先犯肺,未能正确治疗则易逆传心包。 Wind-warm pathogens first attack the lung, and the pericardium may be involved owing to improper treatment.

风消 [fēng xiāo] emaciation due to wind

风心病 [fēng xīn bìng] rheumatic heart disease

风油精 [fēng yóu jīng] essential balm

风雨不节 [fēng yǔ bù jié] failure of wind and rain to come at the right time

风疹 [fēng zhěn] rubella ~ 病毒 virus of rubella/ ~ 块 rubella/ ~ 部位游走不定 German measles spreads rapidly.

风中经络 [fēng zhòng jīng luò] meridians attacked by wind

封 fēng

封闭疗法 [fēng bì liáo fǎ] block therapy

封闭式训练 [fēng bì shì xùn liàn] closed-door training

封藏 [fēng cáng] storage ~ 失职 dysfunction in essence storage

锋 fēng

锋针 [fēng zhēn] lance needle ~ ,可作

为刺络放血之用。A lance needle is used for bloodletting.

缝 féng

缝合［féng hé］sewing up ~ 伤口 stitching a wound

麸敷伏扶服浮福抚俯釜辅腑腐复副腹妇 FU

麸 fū

麸皮［fū pí］bran ~ 面包 brown bread

敷 fū

敷贴［fū tiē］application ~ 药 topical application of herbal medicament

伏 fú

伏案工作［fú àn gōng zuò］sedentary profession

伏脉［fú mài］hidden pulse

伏气［fú qì］insidious pathogenic factor ~ 伤寒 cold-induced disease caused by insidious pathogenic factors/ ~ 温病 warm-pathogen disease due to latent factors.

伏热［fú rè］latent heat ~ 在里 latent heat in the interior/ ~ 指温病中的一种伏邪。Latent heat points to one of the incubative pathogenic factors in a warm-pathogen disease.

伏暑［fú shǔ］latent summer-heat

伏天［fú tiān］dog days

扶 fú

扶阳［fú yáng］strengthening yang ~ 学派 School of Strengthening Yang/ ~ 固表 strengthening yang to secure the superficial resistance/ ~ 固脱 strengthening yang to prevent collapse

扶正［fú zhèng］reinforcing healthy qi ~ 祛邪。reinforcing healthy qi to eliminate pathogenic factors

服 fú

服气［fú qì］taking qi ~ 是通过吸气、咽气等进行的练功方法。In qigong exercise taking qi means breathing in and swallowing qi.

服石［fú shí］taking minerals 在古代，有些修道的人会 ~ 。In ancient China, some Taoists preferred to take minerals.

服药百裹，不如独卧［fú yào bǎi guǒ, bù rú dú wò］Rather than taking a lot of tonics, it's better to rest in bed alone.

服药食忌［fú yào shí jì］avoiding some food in the course of medication

服药时间［fú yào shí jiān］timing of medicine taking

浮 fú

浮沉［fú chén］going up and down; floating pulse and deep pulse

浮刺［fú cì］superficial needling ~ 为古刺法 The superficial needling is an ancient technique of acupuncture.

浮络［fú luò］superficial collateral

浮脉［fú mài］floating pulse ~ 多主表证。Floating pulse often suggests an exterior pattern.

浮肿［fú zhǒng］dropsy 两腿 ~ being

dropsical in both legs/失眠使她眼皮
~。Loss of sleep bagged her eyes.

福 fú

福如东海,寿比南山[fú rú dōng hǎi,
shòu bǐ nán shān] May you have a
long and joyful life.

福寿双全[fú shòu shuāng quán]
enoying both happiness and longevity

抚 fǔ

抚琴[fǔ qín] playing musical instruments
~养生 health preservation with
musical instrument playing

俯 fǔ

俯卧撑[fǔ wò chēng] press-up 练20
次~。Do 20 press-ups.

釜 fǔ

釜沸脉[fǔ fèi mài] bubble-rising pulse

辅 fǔ

辅药[fǔ yào] adjuvant medicinals

辅助手法[fǔ zhù shǒu fǎ] auxiliary
manipulation

腑 fǔ

腑会[fǔ huì] influential acupoint of the
fu-organs 中脘穴又被称为~。
Zhongwan（CV 12）is also known as
an influenctial acupoint of the *fu*-
organs.

腐 fǔ

腐苔[fǔ tāi] curdy fur ~多由食积肠胃
所致。Curdy fur is usually due to
retention of food in the intestine and
stomach.

复 fù

复方[fù fāng] compound formula ~的

效果常常好于单味药。The curative
effect of a compound formula is better
than that of a single medicinal.

复合手法[fù hé shǒu fǎ] compound
manipulation 多种手法同时进行的
推拿方法为~。The compound
manipulations are those used together
in *tuina*-massage.

复气[fù qì] retaliatory qi

复诊[fù zhěn] return visit ~从病人的
病情可知初诊药效。From the
condition of a return visit, one may
know the effect of the medicaments
prescribed at the first visit.

副 fù

副作用[fù zuò yòng] side effect

腹 fù

腹[fù] abdomen 大~upper abdomen/
小~lower abdomen/少~outer part of
the lower abdomen

腹八分[fù bā fēn] eating 80% fill 用
餐最好~。You had better to eat
80% fill.

腹本喜暖[fù běn xǐ nuǎn] abdomen
favoring warmth

腹满[fù mǎn] abdominal fullness ~食
不化 abdominal fullness due to
indigestion/~食减 abdominal
fullness with poor appetite

腹式呼吸[fù shì hū xī] abdominal
respiration ~训练 abdominal
respiration training/顺~orthodromic
abdominal respiration/逆~antidromic
abdominal respiration/~治咳嗽。

Abdominal respiration cures coughing.

腹宜常摩［fù yí cháng mó］massaging the abdomen often ~ 有利消化。 Massaging the abdomen often is good for digestion.

腹中硬块［fù zhōng yìng kuài］hard mass in the abdomen

妇 **fù**

妇科［fù kē］gynecology

妇女病［fù nǚ bìng］woman troubles

妇婴［fù yīng］women and infants ~ 保健 health and fitness for women and infants

G

甘疳肝干感 GAN

甘 **gān**

甘［gān］sweet 甘草性平味 ~ *Gancao*（Licorice）is neutral in nature and sweet in flavor.

甘寒清热［gān hán qīng rè］clearing heat with medicinals sweet in flavor and cold in property

甘寒生津［gān hán shēng jīn］promoting generation of body fluids with medicinals sweet in flavor and cold in property ~ 为润燥法之一。Promoting generation of body fluids with medicinals sweet in flavor and cold in property is a way to remove dryness.

甘寒滋润［gān hán zī rùn］nourishing and moistening with medicinals sweet in flavor and cold in property

甘和［gān hé］（medicinals or food）sweet in flavor and mild in property

甘其食［gān qí shí］satisfied with any food

甘入脾［gān rù pí］sweet flavor acting on the spleen

甘温除大热［gān wēn chú dà rè］eliminating high fever with medicinals sweet in flavor and warm in property ~ 多用于气虚发热、产后或劳倦内伤发热。Medicinals sweet in flavor and warm in property are usually administered to treat fever due to deficiency of qi, internal injury from childbirth or overwork.

甘以缓之［gān yǐ huǎn zhī］medicinals sweet in flavor for relieving spasm and pain

疳 **gān**

疳积［gān jī］infantile malnutrition

肝 **gān**

肝［gān］liver ~ 气 liver-qi/ ~ 火 liver-fire/ ~ 血 liver-blood

肝病禁辛［gān bìng jìn xīn］pungent

flavor abstained in patients with liver problems

肝藏魂[gān cáng hún] ethereal soul stored in the liver

肝藏血[gān cáng xuè] blood stored in the liver

肝乘脾 [gān chéng pí] spleen overwhelmed by the liver

肝胆湿热[gān dǎn shī rè] dampness-heat in the liver and gallbladder ~ 黄疸 jaundice due to dampness-heat in the liver and gallbladder

肝风内动[gān fēng nèi dòng] stirring of liver-wind

肝火炽盛[gān huǒ chì shèng] intense liver-fire

肝火犯肺[gān huǒ fàn fèi] invasion of the lung by liver-fire ~ 可见咳嗽、两肋痛。Invasion of the lung by liver-fire leads to coughing and hypochondrial pain.

肝经[gān jīng] Liver Meridian

肝经湿热[gān jīng shī rè] dampness-heat in the Liver Meridian

肝开窍于目[gān kāi qiào yú mù] eye, the window of the liver

肝咳 [gān ké] coughing with hypochondrial pain

肝脾不和[gān pí bù hé] disharmony between the liver and spleen

肝气不和[gān qì bù hé] disturbance of liver-qi

肝气犯胃[gān qì fàn wèi] invasion of the stomach by liver-qi

肝肾同源[gān shèn tóng yuán] liver and kidney being of the same source

肝肾阴虚[gān shèn yīn xū] deficiency of liver-yin and kidney-yin

肝失条达[gān shī tiáo dá] failure of liver-qi to flow and spread smoothly ~ 则易引起肝郁气滞。Failure of liver-qi to flow and spread smoothly usually leads to stagnation of liver-qi.

肝胃不和[gān wèi bù hé] disharmony between the liver and stomach

肝阳化风[gān yáng huà fēng] wind transformed from liver-yang

肝阳化火 [gān yáng huà huǒ] fire transformed from liver-yang

肝阳上亢 [gān yáng shàng kàng] hyperactivity of liver-yang

肝硬化[gān yìng huà] cirrhosis

肝痈[gān yōng] liver abscess

肝与胆相表里[gān yǔ dǎn xiāng biǎo lǐ] interior-exterior relationship between the liver and gallbladder

肝郁脾虚[gān yù pí xū] stagnation of liver-qi and deficiency in the spleen

肝主筋[gān zhǔ jīn] tendons governed by the liver

肝主谋虑[gān zhǔ móu lù] strategy and tactic governed by the liver

肝主目[gān zhǔ mù] eyes governed by the liver

肝主疏泄[gān zhǔ shū xiè] smooth flow controlled by the liver

干 gān

干呕[gān ǒu] retching ~ 呃逆是由胃

气上逆所致。Retching and hiccupping are caused by adverse rise of stomach-qi.

干热[gān rè] dry and hot ~ 天气 dry and hot weather

干眼症[gān yǎn zhèng] xerophthalmia ~ 可由肝肾阴虚导致。Xerophthalmia is caused by yin deficiency of the liver and kidney.

干支[gān zhī] Heavenly Stems and Earthly Branches ~ 纪年 years designated by the Heavenly Stems and Earthly Branches/中国过去用 ~ 纪年。China used to designate the years by the ten Heavenly Stems and twelve Earthly Branches.

感 gǎn

感官[gǎn guān] sensory organ

感情[gǎn qíng] feeling 复杂的 ~ mixed feelings/伤 ~ hurting someone's feelings

感染[gǎn rǎn] infection 上呼吸道 ~ infection of the upper respiratory tract

刚肛 GANG

刚 gāng

刚柔相济[gāng róu xiāng jì] coordination between yin and yang; coupling hardness with softness; combining vigor and suppleness

肛 gāng

肛裂[gāng liè] anal fissure

肛瘘[gāng lòu] anal fistula

肛门重坠[gāng mén zhòng zhuì] feeling of weight in the anus

肛痈[gāng yōng] anal abscess

高膏 GAO

高 gāo

高埠[gāo bù] mound 居 ~ 者寿。People living on a mound enjoy longevity.

高龄[gāo líng] advanced age, venerable age

高下不相慕[gāo xià bù xiāng mù] not envious of rank and hierarchy

膏 gāo

膏肓[gāo huāng] cardio-diaphragmatic interspace; Gaohuang (BL 43) 病入 ~ disease beyond cure

膏剂[gāo jì] syrup; plaster

膏粱厚味[gāo liáng hòu wèi] fat rich food 长期食用 ~ 易引起肥胖。Long time consumption of fat rich food may lead to obesity. /体胖之人,多有痰湿,则不宜多食 ~ 。It is improper for obese people to have more fat rich food because they are almost suffering from phlegm-dampness.

膏淋[gāo lìn] chylous stranguria

膏摩[gāo mó] ointment rubbing

膏人[gāo rén] obese person with loose skin

膏药[gāo yào] plaster ~ 疗法 plaster therapy

膏滋[gáo zī] soft extract

G

歌割革格隔 GE

歌 gē

歌唱［gē chàng］singing ~ 养生 health preservation with singing

割 gē

割治疗法［gē zhì liáo fǎ］incision therapy

革 gé

革脉［gé mài］tympanic pulse

格 gé

格阳［gé yáng］rejecting yang

格阴［gé yīn］rejecting yin

隔 gé

隔姜灸［gé jiāng jiǔ］ginger-padded moxibustion

隔蒜灸［gé suàn jiǔ］garlic-padded moxibustion

隔物灸［gé wù jiǔ］indirect moxibustion

隔盐炎［gé yán jiǔ］moxibustion with salt

根 GEN

根 gēn

根结［gēn jié］starting and terminal acupoint

弓功攻宫 GONG

弓 gōng

弓箭步［gōng jiàn bù］forward lunge 左 ~ left forward lunge/ ~ 桩 forward lunge stance/ ~ 压腿 forward lunge and flexing one's leg muscles

功 gōng

功夫茶［gōng fu chá］kung fu tea; elaborately prepared tea

功能复位［gōng néng fù wèi］functional restoration

攻 gōng

攻补兼施［gōng bǔ jiān shī］simultaneous elimination and reinforcement 虚实夹杂证用 ~ 法。Simultaneous elimination and reinforcement are adopted to treat a deficiency pattern intermingled with an excess pattern.

攻毒［gōng dú］counteracting toxic substance ~ 扶正 counteracting toxic substances and strengthening healthy qi/ ~ 去邪 counteracting toxic substances to eliminate pathogenic factors/ ~ 杀虫 counteracting toxic substances to kill parasites

攻坚散结［gōng jiān sàn jié］breaking hard lumps

攻溃［gōng kuì］inducing suppuration

攻里［gōng lǐ］attacking the interior ~ 解表 attacking the interior to release the exterior/ ~ 不远寒。Medicinals cold in property sometimes are needed in treatment for interior disorders.

宫 gōng

宫寒［gōng hán］cold in the uterus ~ 不孕 sterility due to cold in the uterus/ ~ 腹痛 abdominal pain due to cold in the uterus

佝 GOU
佝 gōu
佝偻[gōu lóu] rickets

孤箍古谷骨蛊鼓固 GU
孤 gū
孤府[gū fǔ] solitary hollow organ, triple energizer

孤阳不生,独阴不长[gū yáng bù shēng, dú yīn bù zhǎng] Neither yin nor yang can ever exist without the other.

孤阳上越[gū yáng shàng yuè] floating of solitary yang

箍 gū
箍围药[gū wéi yào] medicinal paste around a lesion

古 gǔ
古琴[gǔ qín] *gu qin* (7-stringed plucked instrument in some ways similar to zither)

古玩[gǔ wán] antique ~ 商 antique dealer/ ~ 鉴定 identifying antiques/ ~ 市场 antique market/ ~ 收藏 antique collection

谷 gǔ
谷道宜常撮[gǔ dào yí cháng cuō] contracting the anus frequently

谷道宜常提[gǔ dào yí cháng tí] lifting the anus often ~ 可防治痔疮、肛裂等疾病。Lifting the anus often may help prevent diseases like hemorrhoids and anal fissure.

谷气[gǔ qì] food essence ~ 不行 Food essence fails to move/ ~ 长存 storing up essence of food/ ~ 下流 downward motion of food essence

谷肉果菜,食养尽之[gǔ ròu guǒ cài, shí yǎng jìn zhī] It is necessary to eat grains, meat, fruits and vegetables if one wants to enjoy good health.

谷味[gǔ wèi] food taste

谷消[gǔ xiāo] rapid digestion ~ 故善饥 frequent hunger caused by rapid digestion

谷雨[gǔ yǔ] Grain Rain ~ 茶 tea collected on the day of Grain Rain/ ~ 之时应补血益气。It is essential to reinforce qi and blood on the day of Grain Rain.

骨 gǔ
骨[gǔ] bone ~ 极 bone exhaustion/ ~ 牵引 bone traction/ ~ 伤科 orthopedics and traumatology

骨痹[gǔ bì] bone impediment

骨槽风[gǔ cáo fēng] maxillary osteomyelitis

骨度法[gǔ dù fǎ] bone measurement ~ 是量取穴位的一种方法。The bone measurement is a way to locate acupoints.

骨痨[gǔ láo] bone and joint tuberculosis

骨肉[gǔ ròu] bone and muscle; kin

骨痿[gǔ wěi] bone flaccidity

骨针[gǔ zhēn] bone needle

骨蒸[gǔ zhēng] bone-steaming disorder ~潮热 bone-steaming disorder with hectic fever

蛊 gǔ

蛊毒[gǔ dú] disease due to noxious agents produced by various parasites

鼓 gǔ

鼓胀[gǔ zhàng] tympanites

固 gù

固齿[gù chǐ] strengthening teeth 保持良好的卫生习惯是~的重要方法。Maintaining good hygienic habit is an important way to have good teeth.

固定痛[gù dìng tòng] fixed pain

固肾[gù shèn] reinforcing the kidney ~安胎 reinforcing the kidney to prevent miscarriage/ ~缩尿 reinforcing the kidney to reduce dischage of urine.

刮 GUA

刮 guā

刮柄法[guā bǐng fǎ] handle-scraping ~可以有助于加快针刺的得气速度。Hand-scraping accelerates arrival of qi in acupuncture.

刮痧[guā shā] *Guasha*, scraping ~1周2次。Scraping is applied 2 times a week.

关观管灌盥 GUAN

关 guān

关刺[guān cì] joint needling

关格[guān gé] block and repulsion

关门不固[guān mén bù gù] failure to arrest frequent urination and seminal emission 肾虚可致 ~。Failure to arrest frequent urination and seminal emission is due to deficiency in the kidney.

观 guān

观鼻[guān bí] visualizing the nose

观人勇怯[guān rén yǒng qiè] inspecting the strong or weak physique ~,骨肉皮肤,能知其情。Correct diagnosis is obtained by inspecting the strong or weak physique, and the condition of the bones, muscles and skin.

观赏 [guān shǎng] watching and admiring ~艺术 visual art/ ~植物 ornamental plant

管 guǎn

管乐[guǎn yuè] wind music ~队 wind band/ ~器 wind instrument

灌 guàn

灌肠[guàn cháng] enema ~剂 enema/ 食油 ~ enema with edible oil

盥 guàn

盥洗 [guàn xǐ] body washing and cleaning

光 GUANG

光 guāng

光线[guāng xiàn] indoor light, indoor brightness ~过强,或者过弱,都会伤害眼睛。The indoor light either too bright or too dark all harms the eyes.

瑰龟规归鬼癸桂贵 GUI

瑰 guī

瑰宝［guī bǎo］gem 中医是中国人民的 ~。Traditional Chinese medicine is the rare treasure of the Chinese people.

龟 guī

龟背［guī bèi］kyphosis；tortoise back

龟鳖行气法［guī biē xíng qì fǎ］tortoise breathing（respiration）technique

龟息［guī xī］tortoise-like breathing ~ 动功 tortoise-like breathing *qigong*

规 guī

规范 ［guī fàn］ standard ~ 化 standardizing／翻译 ~ standard translation

归 guī

归经［guī jīng］meridian entry

归真返璞［guī zhēn fǎn pú］returning to original purity and simplicity

鬼 guǐ

鬼神［guǐ shén］demons and spirits 拘于 ~ 者,不可与言至德。Do not discuss medical theory with those who are superstitious.

鬼剃头［guǐ tì tóu］part or complete loss of hair

癸 guǐ

癸水 ［guǐ shuǐ］ menses ~ 藏于肾 menses stored in the kidney／~ 属阴。Menses pertain to yin.

桂 guì

桂花酒［guì huā jiǔ］wine fermented with osmanthus flower

桂圆［guì yuán］longan ~ 肉 dried longan pulp

贵 guì

贵贱［guì jiàn］high or low status 不论 ~,所有病人一律平等。Whether he is high or low, all the patients are equal.／~ 贫 富, 各 异 品 理。Inquiring about the high or low status is to know a patient's constitution and character.

贵柔 ［guì róu］ gentleness prevailing over toughness according to Tao's idea

滚 GUN

滚 gǔn

滚法［gǔn fǎ］rolling ~ 治疗项背痛、偏瘫、关节肌肉酸痛 等。The rolling maneuver is used to treat nape pain, hemiplegia, aching pain of joints and muscles.

过 GUO

过 guò

过劳［guò láo］overwork ~ 死 death due to overwork

过逸［guò yì］too easy and comfortable 过 劳 ~ 均 有 害 健 康。Either overwork or too easy and comfortable life does harm to health.

G

H

海 HAI
海 hǎi

海滨［hǎi bīn］seaside ~ 度假 holiday at the seaside

海水浴［hǎi shuǐ yù］sea bathing 洗 ~ going bathing in the sea

含寒汉汗 HAN
含 hán

含片［hán piàn］tablet for sucking, lozenge 止咳 ~ cough lozenge

含漱［hán shù］gargle ~ 中药 herbal gargles

含漱疗法［hán shù liáo fǎ］gargle therapy ~ 主要治疗口腔、咽部疾病。The gargle therapy deals with oral and throat disorders.

含胸拔背［hán xiōng bá bèi］shrinking the chest and straightening the back

寒 hán

寒潮［hán cháo］cold wave

寒从脚下起［hán cóng jiǎo xià qǐ］cold feeling from the foot ~ , 因此保暖需首先从脚部开始。Since cold feeling starts from the foot, it is important to keep foot warm.

寒霍乱［hán huò luàn］cold choleraic turmoil

寒剂［hán jì］formula cold in property 可治疗热症的方剂为 ~ 。Any formula that deals with the heat pattern is the formula cold in property.

寒极生热［hán jí shēng rè］heat generated by extreme cold

寒厥［hán jué］cold limbs due to yang exhaustion

寒露［hán lù］Cold Dew

寒气［hán qì］cold weather; pathogenic cold ~ 稽留 retention of pathogenic cold/ ~ 客于经脉 cold retained in meridians

寒热错杂［hán rè cuò zá］simultaneous occurrence of the cold and heat patterns.

寒热往来［hán rè wǎng lái］alternative chills and fever

寒热温凉［hán rè wēn liáng］cold, hot, warm and cool 秉天气之阴阳而成 ~ 四气。Herbal medicinals contain the four properties – cold, hot, warm and cool, because they are growing in nature and nursed by yin and yang.

寒疝［hán shàn］periumbilical colic due to cold

寒胜则浮［hán shèng zé fú］edema caused by excessive cold

寒湿困脾［hán shī kùn pí］spleen fettered by cold-dampness

寒暑不适［hán shǔ bù shì］unaccustomed to cold or summer-heat

寒暑适［hán shǔ shì］accustomed to cold and summer-heat

寒痰［hán tán］cold-phlegm ~ 阻肺 lung plugged by cold-phlegm

寒温并用［hán wēn bìng yòng］herbal medicinals cold and warm in property prescribed simultaneously ~ 治疗寒热错杂证。Herbal medicinals cold and warm in property are prescribed for the simultaneous cold-heat pattern.

寒温调摄［hán wēn tiáo shè］adaptable to weather change 孕妇、老人、小儿 应当 ~ 。Pregnant women, the aged and babies should be adaptable to weather change.

寒下［hán xià］purgation with medicinals cold in property ~ 热积 purgation with medicinals cold in property to remove heat/肠胃实热可以用 ~ 法。Purgation with medicinals cold in property is adopted for excessive heat in the intestines and stomach.

寒邪［hán xié］pathogenic cold

寒性［hán xìng］medicinals cold in property ~ 药物有清热作用。Medicinals cold in property act to clear heat.

寒因寒用［hán yīn hán yòng］using medicinals cold or cool in property for pseudo-cold pattern ~ 治疗真热假寒证。Using medicinals cold or cool in property is an approach to dealing with the true heat and pseudo-cold pattern. / ~ 为反治法之一。A pseudo-cold pattern treated with medicinals cold or cool in property is one of the paradoxical treatments.

寒欲渐著，热欲渐脱［hán yù jiàn zhuó, rè yù jiàn tuō］wearing more clothes on cold weather and taking off clothes on hot weather

寒战［hán zhàn］tremble with cold 他突然打了个 ~ 。A sudden chill ran over him.

寒者热之［hán zhě rè zhī］medicinals hot in property prescribed for a cold pattern

寒证［hán zhèng］cold pattern

寒滞肝脉［hán zhì gān mài］cold retained in the Liver Meridian

寒滞胃脘［hán zhì wèi wǎn］cold retained in the stomach

汉 hàn

汉方［hàn fāng］herbal medicine, traditional Chinese medicine

汗 hàn

汗不出［hàn bù chū］absence of sweating

汗出［hàn chū］sweating ~ 表和 exterior pattern released from sweating/ ~ 不彻 impeded sweating/ ~ 不 解 no alleviation on sweating/ ~ 如浴 profuse sweating/ ~ 不止，伤精耗气。

Profuse sweating impairs body fluids and qi. / ~ 当风乃生痤痱。 Prickly heat develops from sweating while being exposed to wind. / ~ 恶风为桂枝汤的适应症。 The *Guizhi* Decoction is indicated for aversion to wind while sweating.

汗而发之[hàn ér fā zhī] dispersing by sweating 病邪在肌表，~。 When they reside in the superficial layer of the body, the pathogenic factors are dispersed by sweating.

汗法[hàn fǎ] sweating method ~ 有退热、透疹、消水肿、祛风湿等作用。 The sweating method is used to subside fever and edema, promote eruptions and remove wind-dampness.

汗剂[hàn jì] formula for sweating ~ 多用辛散轻扬之品，不宜久煎。 Since most of them contain those pungent in flavor and rising in property, the herbal medicinals for sweating are advised to simmer for a short time.

汗家[hàn jiā] patient easily to sweat ~ 不可发汗。 For patients easily to sweat it is forbidden to induce sweating.

汗为心液[hàn wéi xīn yè] sweat attributing to heart-fluid

颃 HANG
颃 háng
颃颡[háng sǎng] nasopharynx

毫浩 HAO
毫 háo
毫针[háo zhēn] filiform needle ~ 疗法 filiform needling therapy

浩 hào
浩然正气[hào rán zhèng qì] awe-inspiring righteousness 中国文化，自古崇尚 ~。 Awe-inspiring righteousness has always been upheld by Chinese culture since ancient times.

合和鹤 HE
合 hé
合病[hé bìng] combination of diseases
合方[hé fāng] combined formula
合谷刺[hé gǔ cì] triple directional needling ~ 为五刺之一。 The triple directional needling is one of the five acupuncture techniques. / ~ 用以治疗肌肉痹证。 Muscular pain and numbness may be treated by the triple directional needling.
合会[hé huì] sexual intercourse 产后满百日乃可 ~。 Have sexual intercourse one hundred days after childbirth.
合剂[hé jì] mixture 复方甘草 ~ compound liquorice
合穴[hé xué] He-sea acupoint ~ 位于肘、膝关节附近。 The He-sea acupoints are located near the elbow and knee joints.

和 hé
和而不争[hé ér bù zhēng] trying to

adapt to the changes and not to combat with them

和法[hé fǎ] harmonizing therapy ~ 包括和解少阳、疏肝解郁、调和肝脾、调和肝胃等。The harmonizing therapy includes relieving symptoms from the *Shaoyang* Meridian, soothing the liver and spleen, and regulating the liver and stomach function.

和肝[hé gān] soothing the liver ~ 止痛 soothing the liver to kill pain

和缓[hé huǎn] soothing 药性 ~ demulcent remedy/脉来从容 ~ smooth beating of pulse

和剂[hé jì] harmonizing and releasing formula

和解[hé jiě] harmonizing therapy ~ 表里 harmonizing the exterior and interior

和利[hé lì] harmonic and smooth ~ 难伤 If blood and qi are flowing smoothly, pathogenic factors cannot invade the body.

和气[hé qì] kind, polite ~ 待人 friendly to people/说话 ~ speaking politely

和声[hé shēng] harmony ~ 布局 harmonic plan/ ~ 大调 harmonic major/ ~ 功能 function of harmony

和胃[hé wèi] regulating the stomach ~ 理气 regulating the stomach and its qi/疏肝 ~ soothing the liver and regulating the stomach

和血息风[hé xuè xī fēng] regulating blood to extinguish wind 脑卒中常使用 ~ 之品。Medicinals to regulate

blood and extinguish wind are often administered in treatment for cerebral apoplexy. / ~ 是治疗血虚所致肝风内动的方法。Regulating blood to extinguish wind is a therapy for stirring of liver-wind due to insufficient blood.

和血止痛[hé xuè zhǐ tòng] regulating blood to kill pain

和药[hé yào] demulcent medicinal ~ 可以用治各种不和之证。Demulcent medicinals are used to treat various disorders.

和营敛汗[hé yíng liǎn hàn] harmonizing the nutritive level to check sweating 桂枝汤具有 ~ 的功效。The *Guizhi* Decoction is prescribed to harmonize the nutritive level to check sweating.

鹤 hè
鹤膝风[hè xī fēng] swollen knee

黑 HEI
黑 hēi
黑疸[hēi dǎn] blackish jaundice

黑面包[hēi miàn bāo] brown bread

黑木耳[hēi mù ěr] black fungus

黑苔[hēi tāi] blackish fur ~ 主极热,又主寒盛。Blackish fur suggests intense heat or cold.

黑枣[hēi zǎo] smoked jujube

横 HENG
横 héng
横刺[héng cì] transverse needling

烘红洪 HONG

烘 hōng

烘干[hōng gān] drying over heat 将某些药物放在烘房或烘柜内,可 ~ 药物 而 不 焦黑。 Some herbal medicinals are placed in a bake house or dryer and they are dried, but not burnt black.

红 hóng

红案 [hóng àn] meat or vegetable cooking

红茶[hóng chá] black tea

红绛舌[hóng jiàng shé] crimson tongue

红舌[hóng shé] reddened tongue

洪 hóng

洪脉[hóng mài] surging pulse 阳明热盛证 可 出现 ~ 。 Surging pulse appears in intense heat of the *Yangming* Meridian.

喉后厚候 HOU

喉 hóu

喉痹[hóu bì] laryngitis

喉关[hóu guān] faucial isthmus

喉 痈 [hóu yōng] retropharyngeal abscess

后 hòu

后天[hòu tiān] acquired; postnatal ~ 失调 lack of proper care after birth/ ~之精 acquired essence

后天因素 [hòu tiān yīn sù] acquired factors ~ 可改变人的体质类型。 Acquired factors can change the types of constitution.

后天之气[hòu tiān zhī qì] acquired qi, the qi that is acquired after birth ~ 由 脾胃运化水谷而来。 Acquired qi produces from the essence of drinks and food transported and transformed by the spleen and stomach.

后下 [hòu xià] added near end 煎药 时,薄荷宜 ~ 。 Peppermint is added near end when a decoction is made.

后阴[hòu yīn] anus

厚 hòu

厚苔[hòu tāi] thick tongue coating

候 hòu

候气 [hòu qì] waiting for mild tingling or aching sensation in acupuncture

呼狐糊虎护 HU

呼 hū

呼吸精气[hū xī jīng qì] inhaling fresh air

呼吸气粗[hū xī qì cū] gruff breathing

呼 吸 气 微 [hū xī qì wēi] feeble breathing

呼吸微徐[hū xī wēi xú] quiet and slow breath

狐 hú

狐臭[hú chòu] body odor ~ 多由湿热内郁 或 遗传 所致。 Body odor develops from internal retained dampness-heat or genetic factors.

糊 hú

糊丸[hú wán] pasted pill ~ 黏性大,崩

解时间比水丸缓慢。Since pasted pills are stickier, their disintegration time is longer than that of watered pills.

虎 hǔ

虎口［hǔ kǒu］part of the hand between the thumb and the index finger

护 hù

护理［hù lǐ］nursing ~人员 paramedic

护胸［hù xiōng］chest protection

花滑化 HUA

花 huā

花剥苔［huā bō tāi］geographic tongue ~属气阴两虚。Geographic tongue indicates deficiency of qi and yin.

花茶［huā chá］scented tea 茉莉 ~ jasmine tea/大多数 ~都有理气疏肝、开胃的作用。Most scented tea works to regulate qi, soothe the liver and whet appetite.

花疗［huā liáo］flower therapy 四季 ~ flower therapy in four seasons

花木垂钓［huā mù chuí diào］gardening and fishing ~, 修身养性。Practice gardening and fishing to cultivate oneself.

滑 huá

滑脉［huá mài］slippery pulse ~主痰热。Slippery pulse suggests phlegm and heat in the interior of the body.

滑苔［huá tāi］slippery fur 水饮内停多见 ~。Slippery fur often indicates internal retention of morbid fluid.

滑胎［huá tāi］habitual abortion

化 huà

化不可代［huà bù kě dài］The natural law cannot be replaced physically. ~, 时不可违。Human growth and development process from birth to old age and death, and the harmony and balance of the human body as a self-organizing system cannot be replaced physically, and the pattern of seasonal changes and the cycle of day and night also cannot be defied.

化火［huà huǒ］transforming into fire 寒郁 ~ fire transformed from accumulated cold

化气理水［huà qì lǐ shuǐ］transforming qi and draining fluid

化脓［huà nóng］suppuration 肌肤 ~ dermal suppuration

化痰［huà tán］resolving phlegm ~开窍 resolving phlegm for resuscitation

化饮［huà yǐn］resolving retained morbid fluid

化瘀行血［huà yū xíng xuè］removing blood stasis to promote blood circulation

踝 HUAI

踝 huái

踝［huái］ankle ~浮肿 swollen ankle/ ~骨折 malleolus fracture

缓换 HUAN
缓 huǎn

缓方[huǎn fāng] slow acting formula

缓急止痛[huǎn jí zhǐ tòng] relieving spasm and pain

缓脉[huǎn mài] moderate pulse ~ 主脾虚、湿证。Moderate pulse usually suggests deficiency in the spleen and a dampness pattern.

缓中补虚 [huǎn zhōng bǔ xū] harmonizing the middle-energizer and reinforcing in a deficiency condition ~ 是一种补益脾胃的治疗方法。Harmonizing the middle-energizer and reinforcing in a deficiency condition is an approach to tonifying the spleen and stomach.

换 huàn

换药[huàn yào] change of medicament 服药后病人出现过敏等不良反应,医生应及时 ~。If side effect like allergy occurs after medicine taking, the physician should make modifications to the medicaments in time.

黄 HUANG
黄 huáng

黄茶[huáng chá] yellow tea ~ 是中国特产。Yellow tea is a Chinese speciality. / ~属轻发酵茶类。Yellow tea is a kind of mildly fermented tea.

黄疸[huáng dǎn] jaundice

黄汗[huáng hàn] yellow sweat

黄家[huáng jiā] jaundice patient

黄腻苔[huáng nì tāi] yellow greasy fur

黄苔[huáng tāi] yellow fur

黄痰[huáng tán] yellow sputum

灰挥恢回蛔会恚秽绘 HUI
灰 huī

灰苔[huī tāi] grey fur ~ 而干者,热证。Grey dry fur suggests a heat pattern.

挥 huī

挥发[huī fā] volatilization

恢 huī

恢刺 [huī cì] lateral needling for relaxation

回 huí

回光返照[huí guāng fǎn zhào] short-lived burst of energy before death ~ 为阴阳即将离绝的表现。A short-lived burst of energy before death indicates soon divorce of yin from yang.

回乳[huí rǔ] terminating lactation

回旋灸 [huí xuán jiǔ] circling moxibustion ~ 适用于风湿痛,神经麻痹 等。Circling moxibustion is indicated for rheumatalgia and neuroparalysis.

回阳[huí yáng] reviving yang ~ 救逆 reviving yang to prevent collapse

蛔 huí

蛔虫病[huí chóng bìng] ascariasis

会 huì

会穴[huì xué] influential acupoint ~ 分布于躯干部和四肢部。Influential

acupoints are located at the trunk and limbs.

会厌[huì yàn] epiglottis

恚 huì

恚膈[huì gé] dyspepsia due to stress and strain ~症见饮食难下，中脘满实，大小便不利等。Dyspepsia due to stress and strain is marked by poor appetite, fullness in the stomach, constipation and difficult urination.

秽 huì

秽毒[huì dú] filth 泻下 ~ purgation of filth

秽脓[huì nóng] fetid pus and blood

绘 huì

绘画[huì huà] painting ~ 调情法 sentiment adjusted by painting

昏浑魂 HUN

昏 hūn

昏闭明启[hūn bì míng qǐ] closing the window at dusk and opening it at dawn

昏不识人[hūn bù shí rén] coma 热极生风都表现为高热，~。Generation of wind due to intense heat results in high fever and coma.

昏倒[hūn dǎo] syncope 猝然 ~ sudden loss of consciousness

昏厥[hūn jué] syncope

昏愦[hūn kuì] muddle-headedness

昏瞀[hūn mào] blurred vision

昏蒙[hūn méng] feeling dazed 感受暑湿之邪，头 ~ 不清。One feels dazed when he is exposed to summer-heat and dampness.

昏迷[hūn mí] coma 高热 ~ coma due to high fever

昏睡[hūn shuì] lethargy 脾虚，~ 露睛。Lethargy with eyes half closed indicates deficiency in the spleen.

昏眩[hūn xuàn] dizziness

浑 hún

浑身疼痛[hún shēn téng tòng] general pain

魂 hún

魂[hún] ethereal soul, the moral and spiritual part of the human being 肝藏 ~ ethereal soul stored in the liver

魂静魄安[hún jìng pò ān] spiritual tranquility

魂消魄散[hún xiāo pò sàn] being half dead with fright

活火霍豁 HUO

活 huó

活络[huó luò] activating meridians and collaterals ~ 止痛 activating meridians and collaterals to stop pain/治风寒痹证，宜祛风散寒，~。In treatment for arthralgia due to wind-cold, it is advisable to expel wind and cold to activate meridians and stop pain.

活血[huó xuè] promoting blood circulation ~ 化瘀止痛 promoting blood circulation, resolving blood stasis and killing pain/ ~ 化瘀理气通络 dredging meridians by resolving blood stasis and regulating qi flow/ ~ 疗伤药 blood-activating and traumatic-curing medicinal substances

活血调经 [huó xuè tiáo jīng] promoting blood circulation to regulate menstruation ~, 理气止痛。Promoting blood circulation to regulate menstruation, qi flow and kill pain. / 痛经,经色紫暗,有血块,治宜 ~,温肾固冲。In treatment for dysmenorrhea with dark red menses and clots, it is advisable to promote blood circulation to regulate menstruation, warm the kidney and reinforce the Thoroughfare Vessel.

活血消积 [huó xuè xiāo jī] promoting blood circulation to remove stagnation ~, 散瘀止痛 promoting blood circulation to remove stagnation, resolve blood stasis and kill pain

活血药 [huó xuè yào] blood activating medicinals 瘀血证,宜用 ~ 治疗。In treatment for blood stagnation, it is advisable to prescribe medicinals that work to activate blood circulation.

火 huǒ

火 [huǒ] fire ~ 性炎上 fire characterized by flaming/木 ~ 刑金 wood-fire phase tormenting metal phase / ~生土 earth phase generated by fire phase/ ~ 为水之所胜 fire phase being restricted by water phase

火喘 [huǒ chuǎn] panting due to fire

火毒 [huǒ dú] toxic fire ~ 内陷 invasion of the interior by toxic fire

火罐 [huǒ guàn] cupping jar 拔 ~ cupping

火逆 [huǒ nì] medical malpractice by using heat therapy

火气 [huǒ qì] internal fire 我儿子 ~ 足, 不怕冷。My son is full of energy. He doesn't mind the cold.

火形人 [huǒ xíng rén] fire-featured person ~ 主要病在金行,包括肺、大肠、皮肤等。Fire-featured people often suffer from disorders of the metal phase (lung) manifested itself as problems of the lung, large intestine and skin. / ~ 多养心。For fire-featured people it is important to nurse the heart.

火郁 [huǒ yù] fire stagnation ~ 发之 dissipation for fire stagnation

火曰炎上 [huǒ yuē yán shàng] fire characterized by flaming

火针 [huǒ zhēn] heated needling ~ 烙法 cauterization with a heated needle/ ~ 疗法 heated needling therapy

霍 huò

霍乱转筋 [huò luàn zhuàn jīn] cramp in choleraic turmoil

豁 huò

豁痰 [huòtán] eliminating phlegm ~ 开窍 eliminating phlegm for resuscitation

J

击饥肌机鸡奇积激急疾集脊季忌剂既纪寂 JI

击 jī

击法[jī fǎ] tapping 棒 ~ beating with a stick/侧掌 ~ lateral-palm tapping/拳背 ~ fist-back tapping/掌根 ~ palm-end tapping/指尖 ~ fingertip tapping

饥 jī

饥不欲食[jī bù yù shí] too hungry to eat

饥饿疗法 [jī è liáo fǎ] starvation therapy ~可以治疗某些神经系统疾病。Starvation therapy is used for some problems of the nervous system.

饥寒交迫[jī hán jiāo pò] suffering from hunger and cold

饥伤脾胃[jī shāng pí wèi] spleen and stomach impaired by hunger ~是脾胃失和的病因之一。Impairment due to hunger is one of the causes of the disorders of the spleen and stomach.

肌 jī

肌表[jī biǎo] skin, superficial part of the body

肌肤甲错[jī fū jiǎ cuò] scaly dry skin

肌衄[jī nù] hematohidrosis 气虚 ~ hematohidrosis due to qi deficiency

机 jī

机关不利[jī guān bù lì] inflexibility of joints

鸡 jī

鸡鸣[jī míng] rooster's crow ~ 至平旦 the period from rooster's crow to dawn

鸡胸[jī xiōng] chicken breast, pigeon breast ~ 龟背 chicken breast and kyphosis

鸡眼[jī yǎn] corn ~ 膏 corn plaster

奇 jī

奇方[jī fāng] formula with ingredients odd in number

积 jī

积精全神 [jī jīng quán shén] accumulating essence and keeping healthy spirit ~是养生的重要法则。Accumulating essence and keeping healthy spirit are important principles in health preservation.

积善 [jī shàn] doing good deeds whenever possible ~成德 following a virtuous path/ ~之家,必有余庆。A family that always does good deeds is sure to have abundant happiness.

激 jī

激光针[jī guāng zhēn] laser acupuncture

急 jí

急方[jí fāng] quick-acting formula ~、缓方为七方之一。The quick-acting and slow-acting formulas belong to the seven categories of formula. / ~治急症。The quick-acting formula is for acute diseases.

急救回阳[jí jiù huí yáng] emergency treatment for resuscitation 亡阳证,宜 ~。In yang deletion, it is advisable to give emergency treatment for resuscitation.

急下存阴[jí xià cún yīn] timely purgation to preserve yin 治疗阳明腑实证,宜 ~。Timely purgation to preserve yin is adopted for the excess pattern of *Yangming fu*-organ.

急者缓之[jí zhě huǎn zhī] relieving spasm with relaxation

急者气味厚[jí zhě qì wèi hòu] herbal medicinals with drastic effect tasting strong

疾 jí

疾病[jí bìng] disease 掌养万民之 ~;以五味、五谷、五药养其病。Physicians who want to take care of all people's health have to adopt five flavors of food, five cereals and five kinds of medicinals to cure their diseases.

疾脉[jí mài] swift pulse ~主热盛或邪盛。Swift pulse suggests excessive heat or pathogenic factors.

疾如风雨[jí rú fēng yǔ] as fast as gale and storm

疾医[jí yī] physician

疾疫[jí yì] epidemic disease 季春行夏令,则民多 ~。If there is summer-like weather in the last month of spring, epidemic disease may be widespread.

集 jí

集邮消愁法[jí yóu xiāo chóu fǎ] collecting stamps to remove melancholy

脊 jí

脊[jǐ] vetebra ~柱 spinal column

季 jì

季经[jì jīng] seasonal menstruation ~见于正常女性。Seasonal menstruation is seen in healthy females.

季胁[jì xié] hypochondrium 少腹引 ~痛 pain of the outer part of the lower abdomen with the hypochondrium involved

忌 jì

忌灯烛照睡[jì dēng zhú zhào shuì] switching off light in sleep

忌口[jì kǒu] abstinence, abstaining from some food 服药 ~ abstinence in the period of taking medicaments/饮食 ~ dietary abstinence

忌冷着汗衣[jì lěng zhuó hàn yī] not putting on clothes soaked with sweat

忌热着晒衣[jì rè zhuó shài yī] not putting on sun-exposed hot clothes

忌湿地久坐[jì shī dì jiǔ zuò] not sitting on wet ground for a long time

忌阴室贪凉［jì yīn shì tān liáng］not staying in a cold room to cool oneself

忌早起科头［jì zǎo qǐ kē tóu］not having one's head exposed to cold air in the morning

剂 jì

剂量［jì liàng］dose, dosage ~ 大小 high/low dosage/ ~ 过大 overdose/ ~ 为每天 3 克 in a dose of 3g per day/ ~ 根据病情而定。Dosage depends on the severity of disease.

剂型［jì xíng］types of formulation; dosage form

既 jì

既病防变［jì bìng fáng biàn］prevention of case deterioration

纪 jì

纪岁［jì suì］signifier of years, which means that qi in the Heaven and Earth controls the climate of a whole year

寂 jì

寂寞无为［jì mò wú wéi］Be quiet and take no action.

加家挟夹假瘕甲 JIA

加 jiā

加减方［jiā jiǎn fāng］modified formula

家 jiā

家和万事兴［jiā hé wàn shì xīng］Harmony in the family leads to prosperity in all undertakings.

挟 jiā

挟持进针［jiā chí jìn zhēn］hand-holding needle insersion

夹 jiá

夹板［jiá bǎn］splint ~ 固定 fixation with splints/小 ~ small splint

假 jiǎ

假寒［jiǎ hán］pseudo-cold 真热 ~ heat pattern with pseudo-cold

假神［jiǎ shén］false vitality 病情危重，则出现 ~。In a critical condition false vitality appears.

假苔［jiǎ tāi］stained tongue coating

瘕 jiǎ

瘕聚［jiǎ jù］abdominal mass

甲 jiǎ

甲子［jiǎ zǐ］cycle of sixty years in Chinese chronology

坚肩兼煎减见健 JIAN

坚 jiān

坚阴［jiān yīn］strengthening kidney-yin 遗精症，采用 ~ 治法，坚肾精，清虚热。For seminal emission it is advisable to strengthen kidney-yin, replenish kidney essence and clear heat in a deficiency condition.

坚者软之［jiān zhě ruǎn zhī］softening hard mass

肩 jiān

肩［jiān］shoulder ~ 不举 failure of the arm to raise due to shoulder pain

肩臂功［jiān bì gōng］functional training of the shoulder and arm

肩臂酸痛［jiān bì suān tòng］aching

J

pain of the shoulder and arm

兼 jiān

兼爱非攻［jiān ài fēi gōng］universal love and non-aggression

兼方［jiān fāng］complex formula ~治兼证 complex formula for concomitant patterns/主方与 ~ primary and complex formulas

煎 jiān

煎［jiān］frying；decocting medicinals；decoction 包 ~ medicinals decocted in cheesecloth/ ~ 膏 soft extract/矿石类药物宜先 ~ Mineral medicinal substances should be decocted first.

煎水代茶饮［jiān shuǐ dài chá yǐn］making a herbal decoction taken as a drink 质轻、含易挥发成分之药可 ~ 。Herbal medicinals, light in weight, with free volatility is often made into a decoction taken as a drink.

煎水外洗［jiān shuǐ wài xǐ］herbal decoction serving as a lotion 清热解毒之药既可内服，也可 ~ 患处。Herbal medicinals to clear heat and counteract toxic substances can either be taken orally or used as a lotion applicable to the lesion.

煎药［jiān yào］decocting medicinals ~法 method of decocting medicinals/文火 ~ ，温补之剂多用之。Slower flame is used in decocting medicinals warm and reinforcing in property. /武火 ~ ，轻宣之剂多用之。High flame

is needed in decocting medicinals light in weight with dispersing property.

减 jiǎn

减肥功［jiǎn féi gōng］body-weight-reduction *qigong*

见 jiàn

见微得过［jiàn wēi dé guò］diagnosis made through examining indistinct symptoms and signs

健 jiàn

健齿［jiàn chǐ］keeping good teeth 勤漱口可 ~ 。To keep good teeth rinse the mouth frequently.

健美［jiàn měi］healthy and fit, strong and handsome ~ 体操 aerobic exercise/ ~ 的体魄 strong physique/ ~ 运动 body-building exercise

健脾［jiàn pí］invigorating the spleen ~和胃 invigorating the spleen and harmonizing the stomach/ ~ 补肺 invigorating the spleen and lung/ ~ 化湿 invigorating the spleen to resolve dampness

健脾化痰［jiàn pí huà tán］invigorating the spleen to resolve phlegm 陈皮能 ~ 。*Chenpi* (Dried Tangerine Peel) is effective for invigorating the spleen to resolve phlegm.

健脾祛湿［jiàn pí qū shī］invigorating the spleen and draining dampness ~方剂 formula that invigorates the spleen and drains dampness

健脾疏肝［jiàn pí shū gān］invigorating

the spleen and soothing the liver 肝郁克脾证,宜采用～法。It is advisable to invigorate the spleen and soothe the liver when spleen disorder is due to stagnancy of liver-qi.

健脾消食[jiàn pí xiāo shí] invigorating the spleen to promote digestion 木香能行气止痛,～。 Muxiang (Common Aucklandia Root) acts to move qi, kill pain and invigorate the spleen to promote digestion.

健脾养心[jiàn pí yǎng xīn] invigorating the spleen and nourishing the heart ～法,适应心脾两虚证。In treatment for deficiency in the heart and spleen it is advisable to invigorate the spleen and nourish the heart.

健脾益气[jiàn pí yì qì] invigorating the spleen and reinforcing qi 脾气虚、中气下陷诸证,宜～法治疗。It is advisable to invigorate the spleen and reinforce qi in treatment for such patterns as deficiency of spleen-qi and sinking of qi of the middle-energizer.

健身球[jiàn shēn qiú] fitness ball

健胃[jiàn wèi] invigorating the stomach ～降逆 invigorating the stomach to descend adversely risen qi

姜降绛 JIANG
姜 jiāng
姜制[jiāng zhì] processed with ginger ～半夏 Banxia (Pinellia Tuber) processed with ginger

降 jiàng
降法[jiàng fǎ] descendent method 升～ ascendent and descendent methods

降剂[jiàng jì] formula with the downward action

降逆[jiàng nì] bringing adversely risen qi downward ～止咳 bringing adversely risen qi downward to relieve coughing/～平喘 bringing adversely risen qi downward to stop panting

降逆化痰[jiàng nì huà tán] descending adversely risen stomach-qi to resolve phlegm

降逆止呕[jiàng nì zhǐ ǒu] descending adversely risen stomach-qi to stop vomiting

降气[jiàng qì] descending adversely risen qi ～药 herbal medicinals working to descend adversely risen qi/～止咳平喘 descending adversely risen qi to relieve coughing and panting

降气化痰[jiàng qì huà tán] descending adversely risen qi to resolve phlegm

绛 jiàng
绛舌[jiàng shé] crimson tongue

交胶焦角绞矫脚 JIAO
交 jiāo
交媾[jiāogòu] having sexual intercourse ～有度 moderated sexual life

交接之道[jiāo jiē zhī dào] principle in sexual life

交司时刻[jiāo sī shí kè] governing the

period of the five dominations in circuit

胶 jiāo

胶囊［jiāo náng］capsule ~ 剂型 capsule form/紫河车粉 ~ Placenta Capsule

焦 jiāo

焦原［jiāo yuán］gate of life

角 jiǎo

角法［jiǎo fǎ］horn cupping

角弓反张［jiǎo gōng fǎn zhāng］opisthotonus

绞 jiǎo

绞肠痧［jiǎo cháng shā］colicky intestinal turmoil

绞痛［jiǎo tòng］colic 胃脘 ~ colic of the stomach/心 ~ angina pectoris

矫 jiǎo

矫正［jiǎo zhèng］correction ~ 药 corrigent/ ~ 治疗 corrective therapy

脚 jiǎo

脚气［jiǎo qì］beriberi ~ 冲心 beriberi with the heart involved

脚湿气［jiǎo shī qì］tinea pedis

疖节洁结解戒 JIE

疖 jiē

疖［jiē］furuncle, boil ~ 肿 swollen boil

节 jié

节气［jié qì］solar term 二十四 ~ 24 solar terms/顺 ~ ,适寒暑,慎起居。 It is important to adapt oneself to the variation of the 24 solar terms, cold and hot weather, and follow a good lifestyle.

节晚食［jié wǎn shí］eating less at supper ~ 有利于身体健康。 Eating less at supper is beneficial to health.

节欲［jié yù］continence ~ 养生 health preservation by continence/循理 ~ Adhere to reason to control desires. / 放情者危, ~ 者安。 Undisciplined passion causes perils and control of desires results in safety.

节欲保精［jié yù bǎo jīng］restricting sexual desires to preserve essence ~ , 怡养天年。 Restrict sexual desires to preserve essence so as to live out one's years to the fullest.

节欲有方［jié yù yǒu fāng］having a fine way of controlling sexual desires 修道之人 ~ ,故长寿不夭。 Those who are good at cultivating themselves have a fine way to control sexual desires, so they usually live a long life.

洁 jié

洁身自好［jié shēn zì hào］keeping one's purity 艾滋病的大爆发提醒人们需要保持 ~ 。 The outbreak of AIDS reminds human beings to keep their purity.

结 jié

结核［jié hé］tuberculosis 肺 ~ pulmonary tuberculosis

结脉［jié mài］irregular intermittent pulse ~ 往来缓。 Irregular intermittent pulse beats slowly at irregular intervals.

结膜［jié mó］conjunctiva ~ 炎 conjunctivitis

结石［jié shí］calculus, stone 胆 ~ gallstone/膀胱 ~ vesical calculus/肾 ~ kidney stone

结胸［jié xiōng］thoracic accumulation of heat, cold, fluid or phlegm

结阳［jié yáng］stagnation of yang

结阴［jié yīn］stagnation of yin

结者散之［jié zhě sàn zhī］enlarged nodes requiring dissipation

解 jiě

解表［jiě biǎo］releasing the exterior ~ 剂 exterior-releasing formula/~ 祛风 releasing the exterior and removing wind/~ 发汗 inducing sweating to release the exterior/~ 发汗可以用浴法。A hot bath is taken to induce sweating and release the exterior.

解毒［jiě dú］removing toxic substances ~ 剂 antidote/~ 药 toxin-clearing medicinals

解肌［jiě jī］expelling pathogenic factors from muscles ~ 退热 expelling pathogenic factors from muscles to subside fever

解痉［jiě jìng］relieving muscular spasm ~ 祛风 relieving muscular spasm and subsiding wind/ 止痛 relieving muscular spasm and pain

解酒毒［jiě jiǔ dú］relieving alcoholism ~ 药 medicinals to relieve alcoholism

解酒醒脾［jiě jiǔ xǐng pí］neutralizing the effect of alcoholic drinks and activating the spleen

解颅［jiě lú］metopism

解热［jiě rè］subsiding fever ~ 剂 formula for subsidence of fever

解暑［jiě shǔ］releasing summer-heat ~ 药 medicinals to release summer-heat/清热 ~ clearing summer-heat

解索脉［jiě suǒ mài］untwining rope pulse

解郁［jiě yù］removing stagnated qi 舒肝 ~ promoting smooth flow of liver-qi to soothe the liver

戒 jiè

戒得［jiè dé］never caring about gaining

戒斗［jiè dòu］avoidinga fight

戒怒［jiè nù］abstinence from anger ~ 是修德的具体体现。Restraining anger is a concrete manifestation of cultivating morality.

戒色［jiè sè］abstinence from sexual desire 少时血气未定，须 ~。Teenagers are usually not vigorous enough, so they have to abstain from sexual desires.

戒烟［jiè yān］quitting smoking 大量研究证据表明，~ 可降低或消除吸烟导致的健康危害。A good number of researches indicated that quitting smoking would decrease or eliminate the damage to health caused by smoking.

金津筋紧谨尽进近浸禁 JIN

金 jīn

金津玉液［jīn jīn yù yè］precious saliva

J

J

金盘玉食 [jīn pán yù shí] luxurious food

金破不鸣 [jīn pò bù míng] hoarseness due to lung dysfunction ~ 常见于晚期肺结核病。Hoarseness due to lung dysfunction is usually found at the late stage of pulmonary tuberculosis.

金伤 [jīn shāng] incised wound

金实不鸣 [jīn shí bù míng] Hoarseness due to attack by external pathogenic factors

金水相生 [jīn shuǐ xiāng shēng] mutual influence between the metal phase (lung) and water phase (kidney) 在补养肾阴时可选用补肺阴的药物，这叫 ~。Medicinals for replenishing lung-yin are used to nourish kidney-yin, which is known as mutual influence between the metal phase (lung) and water phase (kidney).

金形人 [jīn xíng rén] metal-featured person ~ 多养阴润肺。It is essential to replenish yin and moisten the lung for metal-featured people.

金针 [jīn zhēn] gold or metal needle ~ 拨障 cataractopiesis with a metal needle

津 jīn

津 [jīn] body fluid; saliva; sweat ~ 血同源 Body fluids and blood are of the same source.

津枯肠燥 [jīn kū cháng zào] exhaustion of body fluids and dryness of intestines ~，大便秘结。Exhaustion of body fluids and dryness of intestines lead to constipation.

津亏热结 [jīn kuī rè jié] deficit of body fluids and heat retention

津气并补 [jīn qì bìng bǔ] reinforcing body fluids and qi ~ 法适合于气津两亏之证。Reinforcement of body fluids and qi is adopted when there is deficiency of qi and body fluids.

津气亏虚 [jīn qì kuī xū] deficiency of body fluids and qi ~ 多见于久病后，温热病后。Deficiency of body fluids and qi is usually found in patients after a protracted disease or with warm-pathogen disease. /西洋参补气养阴，可治疗 ~。*Xiyangshen* (American Ginseng) acts to reinforce qi and yin, indicated for deficiency of body fluids and qi.

津气两伤 [jīn qì liǎng shāng] impairment of both body fluids and qi

津脱 [jīn tuō] exhaustion of body fluids ~ 者，腠理开，汗大泄。Exhaustion of body fluids leads to looseness of muscular interstices and profuse sweating.

津液 [jīn yè] body fluid

津宜常咽 [jīn yí cháng yàn] swallowing saliva often ~ 可以帮助消化。Digestion is promoted by swallowing saliva often.

筋 jīn

筋 [jīn] sinew, tendon ~ 痹 tendinous spasm with pain / ~ 弛软 flaccidity and weakness of tendons and muscles/~断 rupture of tendons and muscles/~断伤 lacerated wound of tendons and muscles

筋挛[jīn luán] muscular spasm 风动~ muscular spasm due to stirring of wind

筋痿[jīn wěi] muscular flaccidity

筋正[jīn zhèng] soft tissue restoration

筋纵[jīn zòng] flaccidity of muscles and tendons

紧 jǐn

紧唇[jǐn chún] lockjaw

紧喉（风）[jǐn hóu（fēng）] acute laryngeal infection

紧脉[jǐn mài] tight pulse 浮~floating, tight pulse

谨 jǐn

谨察阴阳所在而调之[jǐn chá yīn yáng suǒ zài ér tiáo zhī] Observe yin and yang and regulate them.

谨道如法[jǐn dào rú fǎ] strictly following the law of health preservation ~，万举万全。Strictly following the therapeutic principles ensures successful treatment.

谨和五味[jǐn hé wǔ wèi] having a wise and reasonable allocation of the five flavors of food

尽 jìn

尽终其天年[jìn zhōng qí tiān nián] enjoying good health and long life

进 jìn

进食宜缓[jìn shí yí huǎn] eating slowly

进食宜乐[jìn shí yí lè] having meals in good mood ~有利于消化。Having meals in good mood promotes digestion.

进针[jìn zhēn] needle insertion 单手~法 inserting a needle with one hand/双手~法 inserting a needle with both hands/指切~法 inserting a needle with the aid of the finger of the pressing hand/夹针管~法 inserting a needle with a guide tube

近 jìn

近部取穴[jìn bù qǔ xué] selection of adjacent acupoints 临症时，~和远部取穴可以结合应用，以加强疗效。In clinical practice, selection of nearby acupoints combined with distant ones improves the therapeutic effect.

近视[jìn shì] nearsightedness ~眼 myopia/假性~pseudomyopia

浸 jìn

浸膏[jìn gāo] soft extract

浸剂[jìn jì] infusion 水~water infusion/药液~medicinal infusion

浸酒[jìn jiǔ] medicated wine（liquor）

浸滤[jìn lù] leaching

浸泡[jìn pào] immersion 酒中~immersion in alcohol/水中~immersion in water/药物~medicinal immersion

浸润[jìn rùn] immersion

浸渍[jìn zì] immersion; maceration ~法 maceration/~液 maceration extract

禁 jìn

禁方[jìn fāng] secret remedy

禁忌[jìn jì] contraindicating ~某种药物 contraindicating a drug/食物 ~ food abstinence/妊娠 ~ contraindication in pregnancy/~症 contraindication/汗法 ~ forbidden to use the sweating method

禁声色[jìn shēng sè] abstaining sensual pleasures

经惊粳精颈静镜净 JING

经 jīng

经闭[jīng bì] amenorrhea 气血虚 ~ amenorrhea due to deficiency of qi and blood/血瘀 ~ amenorrhea due to stagnation of blood

经别[jīng bié] divergent meridian 十二 ~ 12 divergent meridians/六阴经的 ~则注入与其表里相合的阳经。 The divergent meridians of the six yin meridians enter the relevant yang meridians which are exteriorly and interiorly related.

经迟[jīng chí] late periods

经断[jīng duàn] menopause

经方[jīng fāng] classic formula ~派 School of the Classic Formula

经筋[jīng jīn] meridian sinew 十二 ~ 具有联缀四肢关节,维络周身,主司关节运动的作用。 The twelve meridian sinews function to link up with the joints of the limbs and dominate their movement.

经绝[jīng jué] menopause 七七天癸竭, ~。 At the age of 49 sex-stimulating essence exhausts and menopause develops.

经络[jīng luò] meridian and collateral ~辨证 differentiation of patterns according to the theory of meridians/ ~敏感区 sensitive area of meridians/ ~现象 meridian phenomenon/通 ~ dredging meridians

经期[jīng qī] menstrual periods ~腹痛 abdominal pain during menstruation

经隧[jīng suì] meridian ~不利 obstruction of meridians/~失职 dysfunction of meridians/五脏之道皆出于 ~,以行气血。 Meridians are the routes of the five *zang*-organs in which qi and blood flow.

经穴[jīng xué] meridian acupoint ~电测定法 acupoint electrometry

经验取穴[jīng yàn qǔ xué] selection of acupoints by experience 以痛为俞, 为 ~ 法。 A tender spot taken as an acupoint is known as selection of acupoints by experience.

经早[jīng zǎo] early periods

惊 jīng

惊[jīng] terror ~厥 faint from fear; convulsion/~则气乱 qi disorder due to terror/大 ~ 失色 turning pale with fright/平肝镇 ~ soothing the liver to relieve convulsion/小儿 ~ 风 infantile convulsion/~悸 palpitation with fear

惊则气乱［jīng zé qì luàn］qi disorder due to terror

惊蛰［jīng zhé］Awakening of Insects

粳 jīng

粳米［jīng mǐ］polished round-grained rice ～牛肉枣葵皆甘。Polished round-grained rice, beef, Chinese date and sunflower are all sweet in flavor.

精 jīng

精［jīng］essence of life ～竭 essence exhaustion/后天之～ acquired essence/先天之～ innate essence/夫～者身之本也。Essence is the root of the human body. /阳～所降其人夭。When yang-qi dissipates, one has a shorter life expectancy.

精满者［jīng mǎn zhě］those with full semen ～不思欲。Those who have full semen don't have sexual desires.

精明之府［jīng míng zhī fǔ］house of intelligence 头又被称为～。The head is also called the house of intelligence.

精气［jīng qì］essence ～内亏 internal impairment of essence/～夺则虚。A deficiency pattern is found when essence is severely impaired. /～日新,邪气尽去,及其天华。Generate essence and expel pathogenic factors, so that one can enjoy a long and full life.

精气神［jīng qì shén］essence, qi and

spirit

精气溢泻［jīng qì yì xiè］experiencing spermatic emission 男子二八,天癸至,～。For a man at the age of 16, the sex-stimulating essence develops, and he begins to experience spermatic emission.

精神［jīng shén］spirit; vitality ～安宁 peaceful mind/～饱满 full of energy; vigorous/～刺激 great upset/～错乱 mental aberration/～呆滞 lifelessness/～恍惚 being in a trance/～昏乱 delirium/～抑郁 depression/～内守,病安从来? If you keep a sound mind, how can diseases come on?

精食气［jīng shí qì］essence supplemented by qi

精血同源［jīng xuè tóng yuán］Essence and blood are of the same source.

精油［jīng yóu］essential oil 玫瑰～rose essential oil

精瘀症［jīng yū zhèng］semen stasis ～是直接影响男性不育的原因之一。Semen stasis is one of the reasons for male sterility.

颈 jīng

颈椎病［jīng zhuī bìng］cervical spondylopathy ～类型 types of cervical spondylopathy/～的发病率不断上升。The incidence of cervical spondylopathy is rising. /经常伏案工作的人～发病率较高。The incidence of cervical spondylopathy among people who always bend on

J

the desk is higher.

颈椎枕[jǐng zhuī zhěn] cervical support pillow ~ 有助于缓解颈部疼痛。Cervical support pillow helps ease neck pain.

静 jìng

静[jìng] peace and tranquility ~ 立 standing still/ ~ 卧少言 quietly on bed with less talk/ ~ 养 resting quietly to recuperate/ ~ 止 static; motionless; at a standstill/安 ~ quietness/镇 ~ 安神 tranquilizing and calming the mind

静功[jìng gōng] quiescent qigong ~ 多采用意守丹田之法。In quiescent qigong one usually concentrates his mind on Dantian.

静神[jìng shén] quietude of the mind without distracted thoughts

静益寿[jìng yì shòu] long life ensured by a peaceful mind

静者寿[jìng zhě shòu] longevity promoted by a peaceful mind ~ ,躁者夭。Those who have a peaceful mind enjoy longevity, and those who are restless die young.

静中有动[jìng zhōng yǒu dòng] motion embodied in stillness 中医养生要求 ~ ,动中有静,动以养形,静以养神。In traditional Chinese health preservation, it is required to have motion embodied in stillness and static state embodied in motion, from which motion helps keep one's figure well and stillness keeps spiritual health.

静坐[jìng zuò] sitting still; meditation ~ 功 meditation in qigong/ ~ 凝神 meditation/ ~ 养生法 meditation to keep healthy/ ~ 是修养身心的一种重要方法。Meditation is an important method to cultivate oneself.

镜 jìng

镜面舌[jìng miàn shé] mirror-like tongue ~ 为胃气将绝的危候。Mirror-like tongue, a critical condition, indicates stomach-qi is on the verge of exhaustion.

净 jìng

净府[jìng fǔ] urinary bladder

净水[jìng shuǐ] purified water ~ 器 water purifier

炅 JIONG

炅 jiǒng

炅气[jiǒng qì] hot qi

九久灸酒救 JIU

九 jiǔ

九刺[jiǔ cì] nine needling techniques

九窍[jiǔ qiào] nine orifices ~ 不利 stuffy nine orifices/ ~ 不通 blocked nine orifices

九转还阴法[jiǔ zhuǎn huán yīn fǎ] nine changes to restore yin ~ 目的在于使阴精化为气血而濡养于周身。Nine changes to restore yin make yin essence transform into qi and blood, thus nourishing the body.

久 jiǔ

久病[jiǔ bìng] prolonged disease ~者, 邪气入深。Pathogenic factors invade the body deeply in prolonged diseases.

久咳[jiǔ ké] chronic cough ~不已,伤及正气。Chronic cough impairs healthy qi.

久立伤骨[jiǔ lì shāng gǔ] bones injured by long standing ~, 累及腰腿。Long standing may injure bones with the lower back and legs involved.

久视伤血[jiǔ shì shāng xuè] blood injured by long watching 肝开窍于目,人的视力赖于肝气疏泄和肝血滋养,因此 ~。Eye is the window of the liver and the condition of eyesight depends on smooth flow of liver-qi and nourishment of liver-blood, so long watching might impair blood.

久卧伤气[jiǔ wò shāng qì] qi injured by long stay in bed

久行伤筋[jiǔ xíng shāng jīn] tendons injured by long walking

久坐伤肉[jiǔ zuò shāng ròu] muscles impaired by long sitting

灸 jiǔ

灸[jiǔ] moxibustion 艾炷 ~ moxibustion with moxa cones/艾条 ~ moxibustion with moxa sticks/直接 ~ direct moxibustion/瘢痕 ~ scarring moxibustion/无瘢痕 ~ non-scarring moxibustion/ ~ 疮 post-moxibustion sore/间接 ~ indirect moxibustion/隔

姜 ~ ginger-padded moxibustion /雀啄 ~ bird-pecking moxibustion/回旋 ~ circling moxibustion/温灸器 ~ moxibustion with a moxa burner

酒 jiǔ

酒剂[jiǔ jì] medicated wine (liquor) ~多具有舒筋活络之效。Medicated wine works to relax the tendons and activate qi and blood flow in blood vessels ./ ~ 既可内服,又可外用。Medicated wine can either be taken orally or used externally.

酒家[jiǔ jiā] drinker

酒浸[jiǔ jìn] steeping in wine (liquor)

酒气[jiǔ qì] effect of alcohol; alcohol fumes ~盛 powerful effect of alcohol/ ~ 与谷气相搏 combat between alcohol and food

酒曲[jiǔ qū] distiller's yeast 造酒美恶, 全在 ~。Distiller's yeast determines the quality of liquor.

酒送服[jiǔ sòng fú] taken with wine (liquor) 行气活血剂,多以 ~,增强其行血止痛的作用。Herbal medicinals for moving blood and qi are usually taken with liquor to strengthen blood circulation and ease pain.

酒渣鼻[jiǔ zhā bí] rosacea

酒者,熟谷之液也[jiǔ zhě, shú gǔ zhī yè yě] liquor being the liquid produced by fermented grains

酒炙 [jiǔ zhì] herbal medicinals processed with rice wine ~后,增强了

药物行气活血的作用。Herbal medicinals prepared with rice wine strengthen qi and blood flow.

救 jiù

救脱[jiù tuō] emergency treatment for collapse

救阳[jiù yáng] rescuing yang ~固脱 rescuing yang to prevent collapse

救阴[jiù yīn] rescuing yin 养血~ nourishing blood to rescue yin

拘居局菊咀巨拒剧聚 JU

拘 jū

拘急[jū jí] contracture

拘挛[jū luán] spasm

居 jū

居安思危[jū ān sī wēi] maintaining vigilance in peace time

居必择乡[jū bì zé xiāng] choosing good environment for residence

居不容[jū bù róng] not having a serious manner at home 寝不尸，~。Do not sleep with stiff and rigid arms and legs in bed, and do not have a serious manner at home.

居处[jū chù] dwelling ~安静 quiet dwelling/ ~相湿 damp dwelling

居处宜忌[jū chù yí jì] favorable or unfavorable dwellings 中国人很注重~和风水，认为这些会影响运势。Chinese people are much concerned about favorable or unfavorable dwellings and feng shui because they think it may affect the family's fortune.

居经[jū jīng] trimonthly menstruation

局 jú

局部选穴法[jú bù xuǎn xué fǎ] local acupoint selection

菊 jú

菊花枕[jú huā zhěn] pillow filled with chrysanthemum flower ~有祛头风，清肝热等功效。A pillow filled with chrysanthemum flower works to expel wind from the head and clear liver-heat.

咀 jǔ

咀嚼[jǔ jué] chewing ~食物 chewing food

巨 jù

巨刺[jù cì] contralateral meridian needling

拒 jù

拒按[jù àn] worse when pressed

剧 jù

剧毒[jù dú] hypertoxic ~物质 extremely toxic substances/ ~性 hypertoxicity

剧药[jù yào] potent medicament 禁用~ forbidden to give potent medicaments/ ~攻毒。Potent medicaments are administered to counteract toxic substances./孕妇应当严禁使用~。It is forbidden to give potent medicaments to pregnant women.

聚 jù

聚精[jù jīng] preservation of essence ~

在于养气 Preservation of essence relies on qi reinforcement.

决绝厥 JUE
决 jué
决渎之官 [jué dú zhī guān] triple energizer

决生死 [jué shēng sǐ] determining survival or death

绝 jué
绝谷 [jué gǔ] fasting

绝汗 [jué hàn] expiry sweating 胸阳闭阻,胸部刺痛,心悸气短;四肢厥冷, ~ 出。 Expiry sweating is often associated with plugged chest yang and stabbing pain, palpitation, panting and cold limbs. / ~ 则终矣 Death follows expiry sweating.

绝经 [jué jīng] menopause

绝育 [jué yù] sterilization 妇科 ~ 术 gynecological sterilizing operation

厥 jué
厥逆 [jué nì] cold

厥心痛 [jué xīn tòng] pectoral pain with cold limbs

厥晕 [jué yūn] syncope

君皲峻 JUN
君 jūn
君臣佐使 [jūn chén zuǒ shǐ] chief, deputy, assistant and guide medicinals

君火 [jūn huǒ] chief (heart) fire

君药 [jūn yào] chief medicinal ~ 是指方中治疗主证,起主要作用的药物。 The chief medicinal in a formula serves to play the main role among other ingredients.

君主之官 [jūn zhǔ zhī guān] chief organ, the heart

皲 jūn
皲裂 [jūn liè] chap

峻 jùn
峻补法 [jùn bǔ fǎ] powerful tonifying ~ 药 powerful tonics/气血十分亏虚的人需用 ~ 。 Powerful tonifying is applied to people with severe qi and blood deficiency.

峻下 [jùn xià] drastic purgation ~ 寒积 drastic purgation to expel accumulated cold and retained food/大黄为 ~ 药。 *Dahuang* (Rhubarb) is a drastic purgative agent.

J

K

咯 KA
咯 kǎ

咯血［kǎ xiě］hemoptysis 肺有郁热～。Intense heat in the lung results in hemoptysis.

开 KAI
开 kāi

开闭［kāi bì］open and close 眼睑的～ open and close of eyes

开鬼门［kāi guǐ mén］opening the sweat pores ～，洁净府 opening the sweat pores to void the urinary bladder

开合补泻［kāi hé bǔ xiè］open-close reinforcing and reducing method

开窍［kāi qiào］resuscitation 活血化瘀，～醒神 activating blood circulation to remove blood stasis and inducing resuscitation/～化痰 resuscitating and resolving phlegm/～息风 resuscitating and subsiding internal wind

开胃［kāi wèi］whetting appetite ～健脾 whetting appetite to invigorate the spleen/消食～ promoting digestion and whetting appetite

开泄［kāi xiè］dispersion and purgation ～实邪 dispersion and purgation to get rid of excessive pathogenic factors

开郁结［kāi yù jié］relieving stagnation ～通腑泻热 relieving stagnation by eliminating heat with purgatives/～适用于痰热瘀血互结于内之证。Relieving stagnation is a method used to treat internal union of phlegm-heat and blood stasis.

开郁醒脾［kāi yù xǐng pí］relieving stagnation and activating the spleen ～法治疗肝郁脾虚证。Relieving stagnation and invigorating the spleen are applied to treat stagnant liver-qi and deficiency in the spleen.

康亢 KANG
康 kāng

康复［kāng fù］rehabilitation ～疗法 rehabilitative therapy/～医院 rehabilitation hospital/早日～ quick recovery/如果治疗及时，护理得当，则病体～较快。If given a timely treatment and good care, the patient can recover soon.

亢 kàng

亢害承制［kàng hài chéng zhì］harmful

hyperactivity checked and restrained to keep balance

苛科颗咳渴客 KE

苛 kē

苛疾[kē jí] severe disease 从之则～不起,是谓得道。If one follows them, severe diseases will not emerge. This is called the way of health preservation.

科 kē

科学用脑[kē xué yòng nǎo] using the brain scientifically ～能发挥潜能。Using the brain scientifically can realize one's potential.

颗 kē

颗粒剂[kē lì jì] granule ～是中成药的一种剂型。Granule is one of the forms of Chinese ready-made medicines.

咳 ké

咳家[ké jiā] patient suffering from chronic cough

咳如犬吠[ké rú quǎn fèi] dog-barking cough

咳嗽[ké sòu] cough ～失音 aphonia due to cough

咳痰[ké tán] expectoration of sputum ～黏稠难出 difficult expectoration of mucous sputum / ～清稀 expectoration of thin sputum

咳吐脓血[ké tù nóng xuè] expectoration of bloody pus

咳唾[ké tuò] coughing and spitting ～血 hemoptysis

渴 kě

渴不欲饮[kě bù yù yǐn] thirst with no desire for drinks

渴喜冷饮[kě xǐ lěng yǐn] thirst with a desire for cold drinks

客 kè

客气上逆[kè qì shàng nì] upward attack by pathogenic factors

客色[kè sè] varied normal complexion 主色与～ individual's normal complexion and varied normal complexion

客者除之[kè zhě chú zhī] eliminating invaded pathogenic factors

空恐 KONG

空 kōng

空腹服[kōng fù fú] taken on an empty stomach 某些补益药物需～效果更好。Some herbal tonics have better effect if taken on an empty stomach.

空气浴[kōng qì yù] air bath

空窍[kōng qiào] orifice

空调病[kōng tiáo bìng] air-condition disease ～主要表现头晕、头痛、食欲不振、上呼吸道感染、关节酸痛等症状。Dizziness, headache, loss of appetite, upper respiratory tract infection and aching pain of the joints are the symptoms of air-condition disease.

空痛[kōng tòng] hollow pain

恐 kǒng

恐[kǒng] fear ～伤肾 kidney impaired

by fear/ ~ 则气下。Fear makes qi sink.

恐惧［kǒng jù］frightened ~ 而不解则伤精。Essence is injured with persistent fear.

扣口叩寇 KOU

扣 kōu

扣脉［kōu mài］hollow pulse

口 kǒu

口不仁［kǒu bù rén］numbness of the mouth 服用乌头一类的药品过量也会出现短暂的 ~ 。Short-time numbness of the mouth may occur if such medicinals as *Wutou*（Common Monkshood Mother Root）are taken too much.

口不知谷味［kǒu bù zhī gǔ wèi］loss of appetite ~ 属脾胃病变。Loss of appetite indicates a morbid condition of the spleen and stomach.

口吃［kǒu chī］stuttering

口臭［kǒu chòu］foul breath ~ 口烂 foul breath and aphthosis/ ~ 多为胃火炽盛。Foul breath is a morbid condition due to excessive stomach-fire.

口疮［kǒu chuāng］aphtha 复发性 ~ recurrent aphtha

口撮［kǒu cuō］lockjaw

口服［kǒu fú］taken orally ~ 药 peroral medicine/药物可分为 ~ 及外用。Medicaments can be divided into two categories：taken orally or for external application.

口干［kǒu gān］dry mouth, thirst ~ 溺赤 thirst and excreting brown urine/ ~ 心烦 thirst with vexation/ ~ 阳热甚 dry mouth due to excessive heat

口噤［kǒu jìn］lockjaw ~ 不语见于中风病。Lockjaw is seen in stroke.

口渴［kǒu kě］thirst ~ 引饮 thirst with a desire for drinks

口苦［kǒu kǔ］bitter taste in the mouth

口僻［kǒu pì］wry mouth

口热［kǒu rè］feverish sensation in the mouth

口热舌干［kǒu rè shé gān］feverish sensation in the mouth with dry tongue

口水［kǒu shuǐ］saliva 流 ~ drooling

口甜［kǒu tián］sweet taste in the mouth

口眼歪斜［kǒu yǎn wāi xié］wry mouth with distorted eye 中风中经络则先 ~ 。Apoplexy involving meridians is firstly marked by a wry mouth with distorted eye.

口宜勤漱［kǒu yí qín shù］washing the mouth frequently

口罩［kǒu zhào］mask

口重［kǒu zhòng］salty；being fond of salty food 我 ~ ，多放点盐。Just much salt, please, I like salty food.

口中和［kǒu zhōng hé］normal sense of taste

口中苦［kǒu zhōng kǔ］bitter taste in the mouth

口中黏腻［kǒu zhōng nián nì］sticky and greasy sensation in the mouth

口中无味［kǒu zhōng wú wèi］tastelessness in the mouth

叩 kòu

叩齿［kòu chǐ］clicking teeth

叩击法［kòu jī fǎ］tapping examination

寇 kòu

寇帚［kòu zhǒu］having a cleaning-up

苦酷 KU

苦 kǔ

苦［kǔ］bitter ~ 味药可以清热除湿。Herbal medicinals bitter in flavor effect to purge fire and remove dampness.

苦寒清热［kǔ hán qīng rè］clearing heat with medicinals bitter in flavor and cold in property

苦入心［kǔ rù xīn］bitter flavor acting on the heart ~ , 故黄连可清心火。Since bitter flavor acts on the heart, *Huanglian* (Golden Thread) works to eliminate heart-fire.

苦温燥湿［kǔ wēn zào shī］clearing dampness with bitter-tasted and warm-natured medicinals

苦夏［kǔ xià］loss of appetite and weight in summer

苦辛通降［kǔ xīn tōng jiàng］dispersing stagnation and purging heat with medicinals bitter and pungent in flavor

酷 kù

酷暑［kù shǔ］the intense heat of summer

快脍 KUAI

快 kuài

快药［kuài yào］drastic purgative agent ~ 通常用来治疗急症。Drastic purgative agents are usually used in treatment for emergency cases.

脍 kuài

脍不厌细［kuài bù yàn xì］being particular about way of cooking 食不厌精, ~ being particular about food and way of cooking

宽款 KUAN

宽 kuān

宽敞适中［kuān chǎng shì zhōng］a house of appropriate size 养生学对居室的要求以 ~ 为度。A house of appropriate size is suitable for keeping good health.

宽舒［kuān shū］free from worry 心境 ~ having ease of the mind

宽松［kuān sōng］spacious；relaxed；loose-fitting/ ~ 的气氛 free and unrestrained atmosphere/ ~ 的衣服 loose-fitting garment

宽中［kuān zhōng］relieving tight chest ~ 理气 relieving tight chest and regulating qi

款 kuǎn

款待［kuǎn dài］treating cordially 盛情 ~ hospitality/设宴 ~ giving a banquet

狂眶 KUANG

狂 kuáng

狂言［kuáng yán］raving

眶 kuàng

眶［kuàng］eye socket 目 ~ 青紫 cyanotic orbit

揆溃 KUI

揆 kuí

揆度奇恒［kuí duó qí héng］assessment of the normal and abnormal

溃 kuì

溃疡不敛［kuì yáng bù liǎn］persistent ulceration

困 KUN

困 kùn

困乏［kùn fá］weary

扩 KUO

扩 kuò

扩创引流［kuò chuāng yǐn liú］debridement and drainage

扩胸［kuò xiōng］expanding one's chest ~ 运动 chest expanding exercise

L

拉垃腊蜡 LA

拉 lā

拉法［lā fǎ］traction ~ 为正骨手法之一。Traction is one of the bone-setting manipulations.

垃 lā

垃圾［lā jī］rubbish 倒 ~ dumping rubbish/生活 ~ house-hold refuse/建筑 ~ demolition debris/ ~ 分类 refuse classification/ ~ 桶 trash can, dustbin

垃圾食品［lā jī shí pǐn］junk food ~ 有害健康。Junk food is harmful to health.

腊 là

腊八粥［là bā zhōu］*laba* congee（rice congee with nuts and dried fruit eaten on the eighth day of the twelfth month of the traditional Chinese calendar）每年农历十二月初八雍和宫向人们布施 ~ 。Lama Temple gives free *laba* congee to people on the eighth day of the twelfth month of the traditional Chinese calendar.

蜡 là

蜡丸［là wán］wax pill

来 LAI
来 lái

来缓［lái huǎn］slow insertion of a needle ~则烦悗 discomfort caused by slow insertion of a needle

来急［lái jí］quick insertion of a needle ~则安静。Quick insertion of a needle makes the patient calm down.

烂 LAN
烂 làn

烂喉丹痧［làn hóu dān shā］scarlet fever

郎 LANG
郎 láng

郎中［láng zhōng］herbalist

劳痨牢醪老 LAO
劳 láo

劳［láo］overwork, overstrain 房 ~ sexual overindulgence/形 ~ physical exhaustion/ ~ 则气耗 qi exhaustion due to extreme tiredness

劳动养生［láo dòng yǎng shēng］keeping fit by labor

劳复［láo fù］having relapse owing to overwork

劳倦［láo juàn］great tiredness ~伤脾 Great tiredness impairs the spleen.

劳咳［láo ké］consumptive cough

劳淋［láo lìn］stranguria due to great tiredness

劳神［láo shén］being taxing 别为我 ~ 了。Don't bother yourself about me.

劳损［láo sǔn］strain 腰部 ~ lower back strain

劳逸结合［láo yì jié hé］having balance between work and rest

痨 láo

痨病［láo bìng］consumptive disease

牢 láo

牢脉［láo mài］firm pulse

醪 láo

醪醴［láo lǐ］medicated liquor

醪糟［láo zāo］fermented glutinous rice

老 lǎo

老而不怠［lǎo ér bù dài］never idle as one grows old

老而寡欲［lǎo ér guǎ yù］having fewer worldly desires as one grows old

老而弥坚［lǎo ér mí jiān］becoming even firmer in one's conviction as one grows old

老花眼［lǎo huā yǎn］presbyopia 肝肾阴虚, ~ 视物不清。Presbyopia is often caused by deficiency of liver-yin and kidney-yin, marked by blurred vison of the aged.

老化［lǎo huà］ageing; degenerating 血管 ~ 。Blood vessels become degenerated.

老黄苔［lǎo huáng tāi］deep-yellow fur ~主热结。Deep-yellow fur suggests internal retention of heat.

老龄［lǎo líng］old age ~ 化 ageing problem

老年［lǎo nián］old age ~ 斑 age spot/ ~ 保健 health and fitness for the aged/ ~ 病 senile diseases/ ~ 公寓 lodging house for the aged

老气横秋［lǎo qì héng qiū］lack of youthful vigor

老字号［lǎo zì hào］time-honored brand 同仁堂是家喻户晓的 ~。*Tongrentang* is the time-honored brand.

乐 LE
乐 lè

乐而有节［lè ér yǒu jié］moderate sexual activity with pleasure

乐观［lè guān］optimistic ~ 主义 optimism

乐趣［lè qù］delight, joy 生活 ~ joys of life

乐善好施［lè shàn hào shī］happy in doing good

乐知天命［lè zhī tiān mìng］submitting to the will of Heaven and being content with one's fate

雷肋泪类 LEI
雷 léi

雷火神针［léi huǒ shén zhēn］thunder-fire miraculous moxa stick

肋 lèi

肋骨［lèi gǔ］rib

泪 lèi

泪［lèi］tear ~ 窍 outlet of the lacrimal gland/迎风流 ~ tears running with wind

类 lèi

类案［lèi àn］assorted case record

类剥苔［lèi bō tāi］exfoliated fur

类书［lèi shū］reference books with materials taken from various sources and arranged according to subjects

类中风［lèi zhòng fēng］apoplectic stroke

冷 LENG
冷 lěng

冷菜［lěng cài］cold dish

冷淡［lěng dàn］cold 态度 ~ indifferent attitude / ~ 待人 giving someone a cold-shoulder

冷敷［lěng fū］cold compress

冷服［lěng fú］taken cold

冷汗［lěng hàn］cold sweat ~ 淋漓 being wet all over with cold sweat

冷静［lěng jìng］calm 头脑 ~ having a cool head or keeping calm

冷漠［lěng mò］indifferent 态度 ~ indifferent attitude

冷暖［lěng nuǎn］change of temperature 注意 ~ careful about changes of temperature

冷热交替浴［lěng rè jiāo tì yù］alternately cold and hot bath ~ 是一种养生法。Alternately cold and hot bath is a way to keep fit.

冷痛［lěng tòng］cold pain 腹部 ~，得

热则减。Abdominal cold pain is relieved by warmth.

冷饮[lěng yǐn] cold drink

冷浴[lěng yù] cold shower

离里理力立丽戾疠利痢例 LI

离 lí

离休[lí xiū] retiring ~ 干部 retired veteran cadre

里 lǐ

里急后重[lǐ jí hòu zhòng] tenesmus 湿热痢疾，大便赤白，~。Dysentery due to dampness-heat usually manifests itself as passing bloody mucous feces and tenesmus.

里脊肉[lǐ jǐ ròu] tenderloin meat

里虚[lǐ xū] interior deficiency 素体 ~ weakness of the body/ ~ 寒证 a cold pattern due to interior deficiency/ ~ 外感 external contraction due to interior deficiency

里证[lǐ zhèng] interior pattern

理 lǐ

理财[lǐ cái] managing financial matters 善于 ~ having skills in financial affairs

理法方药[lǐ fǎ fāng yào] theories, strategies, formulas and medicinal substances 医生必须懂得 ~。Physicians must understand the theories, strategies, formulas and medicinal substances.

理气[lǐ qì] regulating the flow of qi ~ 剂 qi-regulating formulas/ ~ 和胃 regulating qi flow and harmonizing the stomach/ ~ 健脾 regulating qi flow and reinforcing the spleen

理气化痰[lǐ qì huà tán] regulating the flow of qi to resolve phlegm ~ 治疗气滞痰凝之证。The pattern of qi stagnancy and phlegm retention may be treated by regulating the flow of qi to resolve phlegm.

理气化瘀[lǐ qì huà yū] regulating the flow of qi to resolve blood stasis ~ 活血止痛，用于治疗气滞血瘀证。Regulating the flow of qi to resolve blood stasis, and promoting blood circulation to alleviate pain may be indicated for the pattern of qi stagnation and blood stasis.

理气活络[lǐ qì huó luò] regulating qi flow to activate meridians ~ 止痛，治疗气血瘀滞与经脉的痹证。An impediment pattern due to stagnation of qi and blood in meridians may be treated by regulating qi flow to ease pain.

理血[lǐ xuè] regulating blood ~ 剂 blood-regulating formulas/ ~ 祛风 regulating blood to subside wind/ ~ 散风 regulating blood to dissipate wind/ ~ 养血 regulating and nourishing blood

理中[lǐ zhōng] regulating the function of the middle-energizer 补气 ~ reinforcing qi to regulate the function of the spleen and stomach

力 lì

力不从心[lì bù cóng xīn] beyond one's ability

力气[lì qì] physical strength 没~ lack of physical strength

立 lì

立春[lì chūn] Beginning of Spring

立冬[lì dōng] Beginning of Winter

立法[lì fǎ] working out the treating principle ~ 处 方 making a prescription based on the treating principle

立秋[lì qiū] Beginning of Autumn

立如松[lì rú sōng] standing upright like a pine ~,坐如钟,卧如弓。 Stand upright like a pine, sit firm like a bell and sleep on the side like a bow.

立夏[lì xià] Beginning of Summer

丽 lì

丽日[lì rì] bright sun

戾 lì

戾气[lì qì] epidemic pathogenic factors

疬 lì

疬疫[lì yì] pestilence

利 lì

利胆 [lì dǎn] normalizing the gallbladder function ~ 退 黄 normalizing the gallbladder function to treat jaundice/茵陈可以~。 Yinchen (Virgate Wormwood Herb) acts to normalize the gallbladder.

利尿[lì niào] diuresis ~ 剂 diuretics/ 发汗~法 method to induce sweating and urination/~类药物性味多甘淡 平 或 微 寒。 Herbal diuretics are commonly sweet and insipid in flavor, mild and slightly cold in property.

利尿除湿[lì niào chú shī] inducing urination and removing dampness ~ 剂,适用于水湿壅盛所致的癃闭、淋 浊、水肿、泄泻等证。 Formulas that induce urination and remove dampness are indicated for such disorders as difficulty of urination, stranguria, edema and diarrhea due to internal water retention.

利尿通淋[lì niào tōng lìn] increasing excretion of urine to treat stranguria 浊淋宜用~法。 Increasing excretion of urine is often used in treatment for stranguria with cloudy urine.

利尿消肿 [lì niào xiāo zhǒng] increasing excretion of urine to subside edema ~是治疗水肿的重要 方法。 Increasing excretion of urine to subside edema is an important method in treatment for edema.

利小便[lì xiǎo biàn] inducing urination ~常用于治疗水肿。 Edema can be treated by inducing urination.

利咽[lì yān] relieving sore throat ~ 片 tablet for relieving sore throat/ ~ 消肿 relieving sore and swollen throat

痢 lì

痢疾[lì ji] dysentery

例 lì
例假[lì jià] menstrual periods

怜臁敛脸炼练 LIAN
怜 lián
怜贫惜老[lián pín xī lǎo] feeling pity for the poor and aged

臁 lián
臁疮[lián chuāng] chronic shank ulcer

敛 liǎn
敛疮生肌[liǎn chuāng shēng jī] healing sores and promoting tissue regeneration

敛汗[liǎn hàn] arresting sweating ~ 固表 arresting sweating and strengthening the superficial resistance

敛神定气[liǎn shén dìng qì] keeping a peaceful mind and stabilizing qi 学太极拳须 ~ 。 It is required to keep a peaceful mind and stabilize qi in playing tai chi chuan.

敛阴[liǎn yīn] replenishing and preserving yin fluid

脸 liǎn
脸色[liǎn sè] complexion ~ 苍白 pallor/你今天 ~ 很好。You look healthy today.

炼 liàn
炼丹术[liàn dān shù] alchemy

炼己[liàn jǐ] ridding distractions in *qigong* exercise

炼精[liàn jīng] reinforcing the innate essence ~ 化气 reinforcing the innate essence and transforming it into qi

炼蜜为丸[liàn mì wéi wán] making pills with honey 六味药为末, ~ , 每丸重9克。Powder of six ingredients is prepared into pills with honey, 9g each.

炼气[liàn qì] cultivating qi ~ 化神 cultivating qi and transforming it into vitality

练 liàn
练神[liàn shén] adjusting mental activities

炼虚合道[liàn xū hé dào] reaching the state of nothingness to accord with the universal law ~ 是道家内丹修炼的最后阶段。Reaching the state of nothingness to accord with the universal law is the last stage in Taoist practice of *Neidan*.

良凉两 LIANG
良 liáng
良方[liáng fāng] effective recipe 妇科 ~ effective gynecological recipes/外科 ~ effective recipes for external diseases

良药[liáng yào] effective medicine ~ 苦口利于病。Bitter medicine cures sickness, though it is bitter in flavor.

良医[liáng yī] excellent physician ~ 弗为 failure in cure even by an excellent physician

凉 liáng
凉白开[liáng bái kāi] cold boilded water

凉茶［liáng chá］cold herbal tea 喝凉茶可以降火 Drinking cold herbal tea helps remove intense heat. / ~在广东十分流行。The cool herbal tea is very popular in Guangdong Province.

凉风［liáng fēng］cool breeze ~习习 A cold breeze is blowing.

凉肝明目［liáng gān míng mù］removing liver-heat to improve eyesight ~类药以治疗肝热和风热目疾为主的药组成。Medicinals for removing liver-heat to improve eyesight are composed mainly of those herbs that act to remove liver-heat, wind-heat and eye disorders.

凉糕［liáng gāo］sticky rice cake

凉快［liáng kuai］nice and cool, pleasantly cool

凉台［liáng tái］sun terrace

凉血［liáng xuè］removing heat from blood

凉药［liáng yào］medicinals cold in property

凉意［liáng yì］slight chill in the air

两 liǎng

两神相搏［liǎng shén xiāng bó］combination of the reproductive essence of male and female ~,合而成形。The reproductive essence of male and female combines to conceive a fetus.

料 LIAO
料 liào

料酒［liào jiǔ］cooking rice wine

烈裂 LIE
烈 liè

烈酒［liè jiǔ］spirit

裂 liè

裂纹舌［liè wén shé］fissured tongue

临淋 LIN
临 lín

临床施膳［lín chuáng shī shàn］diet ordered in the course of treatment

临风［lín fēng］facing the wind ~站立 standing against the wind

临街［lín jiē］facing the street 窗户~ window facing the street

临睡前服［lín shuì qián fú］taken before bedtime 安眠药通常 ~。Sleeping pills are usually taken before bedtime.

淋 lìn

淋家［lìn jiā］patient with chronic stranguria ~不可发汗,发汗必便血。For patients with chronic stranguria it is forbidden to induce sweating, if any, hemafecia may inevitably occur.

淋证［lìn zhèng］stranguria

淋浊［lìn zhuó］stranguria with turbid discharge

灵陵另 LING
灵 líng

灵丹妙药［líng dān miào yào］miracle cure 你有什么 ~? What miracle have you got?

灵符[líng fú] magic figures

灵龟八法[líng guī bā fǎ] eight-fold methods of the sacred tortoise ~ 是针灸方法之一。The eight-fold methods of the sacred tortoise are one of the acupuncture techniques.

灵魂[líng hún] soul 创新是改革的 ~。Creativity is the soul of reform. / 教师是 ~ 的工程师。Teachers are the architects of the human spirit.

灵兰之室[líng lán zhī shì] a fragrant room for storing books in ancient times

陵 líng

陵居[líng jū] living on highland

另 lìng

另炖[lìng dùn] simmered separately 人参、冬虫夏草等细料多 ~。Some precious herbs such as ginseng and Chinese caterpillar fungus are often simmered separately.

另煎[lìng jiān] decocted separately 某些贵重药, 为了尽量保存其有效成分, 需 ~。Some precious herbs are decocted separately so as to retain their active principles as much as possible.

留流六 LIU

留 liú

留罐法[liú guàn fǎ] retained cupping

留饮[liú yǐn] persisted morbid fluid retention

留针[liú zhēn] needle retention ~ 拔罐 cupping with needle retention/得气 ~ retaining a needle after arrival of qi

流 liú

流火[liú huǒ] erysipelas on the leg

流浸膏[liú jìn gāo] liquid extract

流食[liú shí] liquid diet

流水不腐, 户枢不蠹[liú shuǐ bù fǔ, hù shū bù dù] keeping things in use, keeping them work

六 liù

六腑[liù fǔ] six *fu*-organs ~ 的特点是泄而不藏。The characteristic of the six *fu*-organs is discharge without storage. / ~ 以通为用。The six *fu*-organs function well when they are unobstructed.

六极[liù jí] six kinds of exhaustion ~ 为极度虚损的病证。Six kinds of exhaustion refer to the extreme deficiency patterns.

六节[liù jié] six restrictions ~ 以养身心。Cultivate oneself with six restrictions.

六经辨证[liù jīng biàn zhèng] differentiation of patterns according to the theory of the six meridians

六气[liù qì] six climatic factors ~ 运行 move of the six climatic factors/ ~ 失常 abnormality of the six climatic factors

六淫[liù yín] six excesses, adverse environmental conditions of wind, cold, dryness, dampness, fire and summer-heat 外感 ~ 邪气 exposure to the

L

adverse environmental conditions of wind, cold, dryness, dampness, fire and summer-heat

六郁[liù yù] six kinds of stagnation 气郁、痰郁、血瘀、食郁、湿郁和火郁统称 ~ Six kinds of stagnation include stagnation of qi, phlegm, blood, food, dampness and fire.

六字诀[liù zì jué] six healing sounds

癃 LONG

癃 lóng

癃闭[lóng bì] difficulty of urination, anuria

漏 lòu

漏汗[lòu hàn] persistent sweating

卤露 LU

卤 lǔ

卤菜[lǔ cài] pot-stewed meat dish

卤面[lǔ miàn] noodles with meat and gravy

卤味[lǔ wèi] pot-stewed meat served cold

露 lù

露[lù] distillate; syrup; juice 草莓 ~ strawberry syrup/玫瑰 ~ rose juice/杏仁 ~ almond juice/药 ~ distilled medicated liquid

露剂[lù jì] distillate ~ 为中药制剂的一种剂型。Distillate is a herbal preparation.

挛 LUAN

挛 luán

挛痹[luán bì] impediment with muscular contracture

罗瘰络 LUO

罗 luó

罗宋汤[luó sòng tāng] borsch

瘰 luǒ

瘰疬[luǒ lì] scrofula

络 luò

络脉[luò mài] collateral

络穴[luò xué] Luo-connecting acupoint 针刺 ~ needling the Luo-connecting acupoints

旅绿 Lǚ

旅 lǚ

旅游[lǚ yóu] tour

绿 lǜ

绿茶[lǜ chá] green tea

绿豆枕[lǜ dòu zhěn] pillow filled with mung bean ~ 可以清热。A pillow filled with mung been helps to clear heat.

绿化[lǜ huà] afforest ~ 城市 making the city green/ ~ 地带 greenbelt

绿色食品[lǜ sè shí pǐn] eco-food

M

麻马 MA

麻 má

麻痹舌[má bì shé] paralytic tongue

麻促脉[má cù mài] rapid and irregular pulse

麻木［má mù］numbness 四肢 ~ numbness of limbs

麻胀感［má zhàng gǎn］tingling and distending sensation

麻疹[má zhěn] measles ~ 不透 measles without adequate eruptions/ ~ 逆证 a severe deteriorative case of measles/ ~ 顺证 measles with favorable prognosis/ ~ 险证 a critical case of measles

马 mǎ

马步［mǎ bù］horse stance 蹲 ~ practicing horse stance

马刀侠瘿[mǎ dāo xiá yǐng] sabre and bead-string scrofula

马桶癣［mǎ tǒng xuǎn］contact dermatitis of buttocks

马牙[mǎ yá] newborn gingival cyst

埋脉 MAI

埋 mái

埋线疗法［mái xiàn liáo fǎ］ medicament-embedding therapy

埋针疗法[mái zhēn liáo fǎ] needle-embedding therapy

埋植疗法［mái zhí liáo fǎ］object-embedding therapy

脉 mài

脉迟[mài chí] slow pulse

脉从四时［mài cóng sì shí］pulse agreeing with seasonal variations ~ 有春弦、夏洪、秋毛、冬石之分。A pulse agrees with seasonal variations, for example, the pulse in spring is somewhat wiry, full in summer, floating in autumn and deep in winter.

脉从阴阳［mài cóng yīn yáng］pulse conforming to the conditions of yin and yang ~，病易已。If the pulse conforms to the conditions of yin and yang, the disease is easy to cure.

脉动无常［mài dòng wú cháng］irregular beating of pulse

脉和[mài hé] normal pulse ~ 是正常人的脉象。Normal pulse is seen in healthy people. ~ 说明有胃气。Normal pulse reflects good function of stomach-qi.

脉逆四时［mài nì sì shí］pulse disagreeing with seasonal variations

脉散[mài sǎn] scattered pulse 元气耗散,脏气将绝, ~ 。Scattered pulse occurs when original qi is dissipated and the qi of the zang-organs vanishes.

脉涩[mài sè] chopped pulse ~ 具有脉律不齐的特点。Chopped pulse is characterized by irregular pulse rhythm.

脉脱[mài tuō] missing pulse ~ ,多见于休克病人。Missing pulse is often seen in shock patients.

脉微肢冷[mài wēi zhī lěng] faint pulse and cold limbs

脉痿[mài wěi] vessel flaccidity

脉细[mài xì] thready pulse

脉弦[mài xián] wiry pulse

脉象[mài xiàng] pulse manifestation

脉学[mài xué] study of Chinese pulse quality, sphygmology

脉诊[mài zhěn] pulse diagnosis

脉证合参 [mài zhèng hé cān] comprehensive analysis of the pulse condition and pattern ~ ,以决死生。With a comprehensive analysis of the pulse condition and pattern, the outcome of a disease is predicted.

慢 MAN
慢 màn

慢惊风 [màn jīng fēng] chronic infantile convulsion

慢性[màn xìng] chronic ~ 腰肌劳损 chronic lumbar muscle strain

芒 MANG
芒 máng

芒刺舌[máng cì shé] prickly tongue ~ 主热证。Prickly tongue suggests a heat pattern.

芒针[máng zhēn] elongated needle

芒种[máng zhòng] Grain in Ear

毛冒瞀 MAO
毛 máo

毛刺[máo cì] skin needling

毛发 [máo fà] hair ~ 枯焦 shrivelled hair

毛孔 [máo kǒng] sweat pore ~ 闭塞 blocked sweat pores

冒 mào

冒家 [mào jiā] patient with frequent dizziness ~ 汗出自愈。Patients with frequent dizziness are self cured by sweating.

瞀 mào

瞀郁[mào yù] dizziness and depression

梅霉美 MEI
梅 méi

梅毒[méi dú] syphilis

梅核气[méi hé qì] globus hysterics

梅花针[méi huā zhēn] plum-blossom needling ~ 疗法 plum-blossom needling therapy

梅雨季节[méi yǔ jì jié] rainy season ~ 食物容易发霉。Food often goes mouldy in the rainy season.

霉 méi

霉酱苔[méi jiàng tāi] rotten-curdy fur

美 měi

美其服[měi qí fú] satisfied with any clothes

美容[měi róng] beauty treatment ～院 beauty salon/中医 ～ traditional Chinese beauty treatment/～正成为一种时尚。Beauty treatment has recently become fashionable.

美食家[měi shí jiā] epicure

闷 MEN

闷 mēn

闷热[mēn rè] muggy 天气 ～ sultry weather

闷 mèn

闷气[mèn qì] sulk 不要生 ～。Do not have the sulks.

蒙梦孟 MENG

蒙 měng

蒙医学[měng yī xué] traditional Mongolian medicine

梦 mèng

梦遗[mèng yí] nocturnal emission

梦呓[mèng yì] sleep-talking

梦游[mèng yóu] sleep-walking

孟 mèng

孟春[mèng chūn] early spring, which refers to the first month of spring

孟冬[mèng dōng] early winter, which refers to the first month of winter

孟秋[mèng qiū] early autumn, which refers to the first month of autumn

孟夏[mèng xià] early summer, which refers to the first month of summer

迷米泌秘蜜 MI

迷 mí

迷睡[mí shuì] deep sleep ～ 不醒 unable to wake up from deep sleep

米 mǐ

米粉肉[mǐ fěn ròu] pork steamed with glutinous rice

米泔水[mǐ gān shuǐ] rice-washed water ～浸药 herbal medicinals soaked in rice-washed water

米酒[mǐ jiǔ] rice wine

米汤[mǐ tāng] water in which rice has been cooked

泌 mì

泌别清浊[mì bié qīng zhuó] separating usable substances from unusable substances

秘 mì

秘方[mì fāng] secret recipe 宫廷 ～ secret recipes of the imperial court/祖传 ～ secret recipes handed down in the family from generation to generation

蜜 mì

蜜煎导[mì jiān dǎo] honey suppository ～用于治便秘。A honey suppository is given to relieve constipation.

蜜丸[mì wán] honeyed pill ～ 水丸 honeyed pills and watered pills/～药

性平和，常用于治疗慢性疾患。Honeyed pills, mild in action, are usually administered for chronic conditions.

蜜灸法［mì zhì fǎ］processed with honey ~ 在中药炮制中应用广泛。Processing with honey is widely used in preparing herbal medicinals. / 百合清心安神，~ 加工后可增加其药效。Baihe (Lily Bulb) effects to clear heart-fire and calm the mind. Its action is strengthened after being processed with honey.

棉面 MIAN
棉 mián
棉织品［mián zhī pǐn］cotton fabrics

面 miàn
面包屑［miàn bāo xiè］bread crump

面壁［miàn bì］facing a wall ~ 修炼 Face a wall and practice asceticism.

面茶［miàn chá］seasoned flour mush

面点［miàn diǎn］pastry made from wheat flour 西式 ~ western-style pastry

面浮［miàn fú］puffy face

面红［miàn hóng］flushed face 肝火上炎则表现为 ~ 赤。Flaming of liver-fire leads to flushed face and eyes.

面黄［miàn huáng］sallow complexion ~ 肌瘦 emaciation with a sallow complexion

面片［miàn piàn］dough strip

面色［miàn sè］complexion ~ 红润 rosy cheeks

面色㿠白［miàn sè huàng bái］pallor ~ 多属阳虚水泛。Pallor and facial puffiness indicate yang deficiency and flooding of water.

面色黧黑［miàn sè lí hēi］darkish complexion 血瘀日久，可致 ~。Persistent blood stasis leads to a darkish complexion.

面瘫［miàn tān］facial paralysis

面宜多擦［miàn yí duō cā］rubbing the face often

面由心生［miàn yóu xīn shēng］facial look revealing the mind condition

面针［miàn zhēn］facial acupuncture ~ 疗法 facial acupuncture therapy / ~ 麻醉 facial acupuncture anesthesia

苗 MIAO
苗 miáo
苗窍［miáo qiào］body opening

苗医学［miáo yī xué］Miao ethnic medicine

灭 MIE
灭 miè
灭孑孓［miè jié jué］killing mosquito larva 除污水以 ~ Get rid of polluted water and kill mosquito larvae.

民 MIN
民 mín
民间药方［mín jiān yào fāng］folk recipe

名明鸣冥命 MING

名 míng

名老中医 [míng lǎo zhōng yī] outstanding senior traditional Chinese medicine practitioner

明 míng

明暗 [míng àn] brightness and darkness 阴阳适中, ~ 相半 balance between yin and yang, appropriate darkness and brightness

明眸皓齿 [míng móu hào chǐ] clear bright eyes and white teeth

明目 [míng mù] improving vision ~ 聪耳 improving vision and hearing/ ~ 退翳 improving vision and removing nebula/清肝 ~ clearing liver-fire to improve vision/枸杞子有 ~ 的作用。 *Gouqizi* (Barbary Wolfberry Fruit) has the effect of improving vision.

明目枕 [míng mù zhěn] eyesight-improving pillow

明堂 [míng táng] nose; acupoint; chart

鸣 míng

鸣天鼓 [míng tiān gǔ] striking the heavenly drum

冥 míng

冥想 [míng xiǎng] meditation 许多忙碌的主管开始练习瑜伽和 ~。 Many busy executives have begun to practice yoga and meditation.

命 mìng

命关 [mìng guān] life gate ~ 火衰 decline of the fire of the life gate/ ~ 之火 fire of the life gate/ ~ 之水 water of the life gate

命门 [mìng mén] life gate ~ 之火 fire of the life gate/ ~ 火衰多是以身体机能减退为标志的。Decline of the fire of the life gate is marked by general hypofunction. / ~ 者,精神之所舍,原气之所系也。The life gate is the house of essence and spirit, and the source of original qi.

缪 MIU

缪 miù

缪刺 [miù cì] contralateral puncture ~ 法可以治疗水肿。The contralateral puncture is applied to treating edema.

摸膜摩抹 MO

摸 mō

摸法 [mō fǎ] palpation

膜 mó

膜原 [mó yuán] space between the exterior and interior 邪在 ~。 Pathogenic factors lodge in the space between the exterior and interior.

摩 mó

摩法 [mó fǎ] rubbing

摩腹 [mó fù] rubbing the abdomen 运气 rubbing the abdomen and moving qi/ ~ 治疗便秘 Abdominal rubbing cures constipation.

摩目 [mó mù] rubbing eyes 热手 ~ rubbing eyes with warm hands/ ~ 能

M

增强视力,防止近视。Rubbing eyes with warm hands improves vision and prevents shortsightedness.

摩腰[mó yāo] lower back massage ~ 有强腰壮肾之功。Lower back massage strengthens the lower back and kidney.

抹 mǒ

抹法[mǒ fǎ] gentle rubbing ~ 具有醒脑开窍、清利头目、平肝镇静、舒筋解痛等作用。Gentle rubbing works to resuscitate, refresh the head and eyes, soothe the liver to tranquilize, and relax muscles and relieve pain.

母拇木沐目募暮 MU

母 mǔ

母病及子[mǔ bìng jí zǐ] disorder of the mother-organ affecting its child-organ

母乳[mǔ rǔ] breast milk 喂养 ~ breast-feeding 她用 ~ 喂养女儿。She feeds her daughter with milk from her breasts.

拇 mǔ

拇食指押手法[mǔ shí zhǐ yā shǒu fǎ] thumb-index finger pressing maneuver

拇指同身寸[mǔ zhǐ tóng shēn cùn] thumb body-*cun* 使用 ~ ,确定穴位位置 locating an acupoint by the thumb body-*cun*

木 mù

木火刑金[mù huǒ xíng jīn] wood phase (liver) and fire phase (heart)

tormenting metal phase (lung)

木形人[mù xíng rén] wood-featured person ~ 主要病在土行,包括脾胃、肌肉等。Wood-featured people often suffer from disorders of the earth phase (spleen-stomach) and muscles. / ~ 应疏脾调胃。For wood-featured people it is essential to regulate the spleen and stomach.

木曰曲直[mù yuē qū zhí] wood phase (liver) being characterized by bending and straightening

沐 mù

沐[mù] washing the head and face

目 mù

目不久视[mù bù jiǔ shì] not staring at something for a long time

目得血而能视[mù dé xuè ér néng shì] good eyesight ensured by abundant blood supply to the eyes 血养目, ~ 。Blood nourishes eyes and good eyesight depends on abundant blood supply to the eyes.

目光[mù guāng] view ~ 如豆 having a narrow vision/ ~ 如炬 with eyes blazing

目昏[mù hūn] blurred vision

目力[mù lì] vision ~ 不济 having poor eyesight

目迷五色[mù mí wǔ sè] being dazzled by a complicated situation

目冥[mù míng] dim eyesight ~ 耳聋 dim eyesight and deafness

目内眦[mù nèi zì] inner canthus

目锐眦[mù ruì zì] outer canthus 丝竹空位于 ~。Sizhukong (TE 23) is located at the outer canthus.

目为肝窍[mù wéi gān qiào] eye, the window of the liver

目眩[mù xuàn] feeling dizzy

目宜常运[mù yí cháng yùn] moving eyeballs often ~,清肝明目。Moving eyeballs often helps clear liver-heat and improve eyesight.

目眦[mù zì] canthus ~痒 itchy canthus

募 mù

募穴[mù xué] Mu-alarm acupoint ~常用于诊断和治疗本脏腑的疾患。The Mu-alarm acupoints are usually used in diagnosis or treatment for diseases in their own *zang-fu* organs.

暮 mù

暮热早凉[mù rè zǎo liáng] fever in the evening and subsidence of fever in the morning 阴虚病人多见 ~。Patients with yin deficiency usually have fever in the evening and subsidence of fever in the morning.

暮无饱食[mù wú bǎo shí] eating less at supper

N

拿纳 NA

拿 ná

拿法[ná fǎ] grasping 三指 ~ three-finger grasping/五指 ~ five-finger grasping/~ 的刺激性较强。The grasping maneuver gives stronger stimulation. / ~是推拿手法之一。Grasping is one of the *tuina*-massage manipulations.

拿捏法[ná niē fǎ] grasping-pinching ~ 属骨伤科治法。The grasping-pinching maneuver is in the range of treatment for fracture and wound.

纳 nà

纳(乘)凉[nà (chéng) liáng] enjoying the cool 人们经常在夏季 ~时焚烧艾草,驱除蚊子。In summer, people usually burn the argy wormwood leaves to expel mosquitoes when enjoying the cool.

纳呆[nà dāi] poor appetite

纳气 [nà qì] grasping qi ~ 平喘 grasping qi to relieve panting

纳正[nà zhèng] restoring to the normal position

奶耐 NAI

奶 nǎi

奶茶[nǎi chá] tea with milk

奶酒[nǎi jiǔ] fermented milk

奶癣[nǎi xuǎn] infantile eczema ~常见于婴儿头面部。Infantile eczema is often found in baby's head and face.

耐 nài

耐高温[nài gāo wēn] high-temperature resistant

耐寒[nài hán] cold-resistant

耐力运动[nài lì yùn dòng] endurance exercise ~能够延长肌细胞寿命,延缓肌肉老化。Endurance exercise may prolong muscular cell's life and prevent the ageing process of muscles.

南难 NAN

南 nán

南豆腐[nán dòu fu] southern-style tofu

南味[nán wèi] of southern taste and flavor ~小吃 southern-style snack

难 nán

难产[nán chǎn] difficult labor

难治[nán zhì] difficult to cure

囊 NANG

囊 náng

囊痈[náng yōng] scrotal abscess

蛲脑臑 NAO

蛲 náo

蛲虫病[náo chóng bìng] enterobiasis

脑 nǎo

脑[nǎo] brain ~疽 nape cellulitis/ ~鸣 humming in the head/ ~震荡 cerebral concussion/ ~卒中 cerebral apoplexy/ ~为元神之府。The brain is the seat of mental activities.

臑 nào

臑[nào] upper arm ~骨 humerus/ ~内 medial aspect of the upper arm/ ~外 lateral aspect of the upper arm

内 NEI

内 nèi

内闭外脱 [nèi bì wài tuō] loss of consciousness and collapse

内丹[nèi dān] *Neidan*, inner elixir ~功 *Neidan qigong*/ ~术 inner elixir art

内风[nèi fēng] internal wind

内功[nèi gōng] inner activity *qigong* 少林 ~ Shaolin inner activity *qigong*

内寒[nèi hán] internal cold

内景[nèi jǐng] inner scene

内科[nèi kē] internal medicine

内廉[nèi lián] medial aspect ~疮 ulcer on the medial aspect

内气[nèi qì] inner qi ~外放 emitting inner qi/修炼 ~ cultivating inner qi/练习 ~的主要方法是站桩和打坐。Stance training and meditation are the chief approaches in cultivation of inner qi.

内热[nèi rè] internal heat 肥者令人 ~,甘者令人中满。Excessive fat food can cause the body to produce internal heat. Excessive sweet food can cause abdominal distension.

内伤[nèi shāng] internal injury ~头痛 headache due to internal injury/ ~发热 fever due to internal injury ~脾胃,百病从生。Multiple diseases are caused by injury to the spleen and stomach.

内湿[nèi shī] internal dampness

内视[nèi shì] inward vision

内省[nèi xǐng] self-examination 见贤思齐焉,见不贤而 ~ 也。On seeing a man of virtue, try to become his equal; on seeing a man without virtue, examine yourself not to have the same defects.

内养功[nèi yǎng gōng] health-building qigong ~是采取一定呼吸法,并配合默念词句的一种气功功法。In practice of the health-building qigong, one has to follow a set of breathing techniques accompanied by reading silently some secret words. / ~具有大脑静,脏腑动的特点。In practice of the health-building qigong one has to calm the mind with dynamic internal organs.

内因[nèi yīn] internal cause 中医把病因分为 ~、外因和不内外因。In traditional Chinese medicine, disease causes are divided into the internal, external, and neither internal nor external causes. /致病 ~ 为内伤七情。The internal cause of disease refers to internal injury caused by seven abnormal emotions.

内燥[nèi zào] internal dryness

内障外翳[nèi zhàng wài yì] cataract and nebula

内针[nèi zhēn] inserting a needle

内治[nèi zhì] internal treatment ~与外治 internal treatment and external treatment

嫩 NEN

嫩 nèn

嫩豆腐[nèn dòu fu] soft tofu

泥逆溺腻 NI

泥 ní

泥丸[ní wán] brain; mud ball; upper Dantian ~ 主元神 Mentality is dominated by the brain.

泥浴[ní yù] mud bath ~疗法 mud bath therapy

逆 nì

逆传[nì chuán] reverse transmission ~心包 reverse transmission to the pericardium

逆乱[nì luàn] derangement

逆证[nì zhèng] unfavorable pattern

溺 nì

溺水[nì shuǐ] drowning 抢救 ~ emergency treatment for drowning

腻 nì

腻苔[nì tāi] greasy fur 黏 ~ sticky and greasy fur

N

捻年 NIAN
捻 niǎn
捻转[niǎn zhuǎn] twirling and rotating 补泻 ~ reinforcing and reducing by twirling and rotating

年 nián
年老体弱[nián lǎo tǐ ruò] being worn out with age

尿 NIAO
尿 niào
尿闭[niào bì] anuresis
尿急[niào jí] urgency of urination
尿血[niào xuè] hematuria
尿浊[niào zhuó] turbid urine

捏 NIE
捏 niē
捏[niē] pinching 三指 ~ pinching with three fingers
捏脊[niē jǐ] spine pinching 小儿 ~ 疗法 spine pinching therapy for children/ ~ 法治疗小儿脾胃虚弱之疳积症。The spine pinching is adopted to treat infantile malnutrition due to hypofunction of the spleen and stomach. /经常给小儿 ~，可以提高小儿的抵抗力。The spine pinching given constantly to children may strengthen their body resistance.
捏眦[niē zì] pressing the inner and outer canthus ~ 防疲劳 Pressing the inner and outer canthus effects to get rid of tiredness. / ~ 有明目作用。Vision is improved by pressing the inner and outer canthus.

宁 NING
宁 níng
宁静[níng jìng] peaceful ~ 的生活 peaceful life
宁静淡泊[níng jìng dàn bó] tranquil and indifferent to fame and fortune
宁心安神[níng xīn ān shén] relieving mental stress
宁心固肾[níng xīn gù shèn] calming the mind and reinforcing the kidney

牛 NIU
牛 niú
牛皮癣[niú pí xuǎn] psoriasis
牛肉[niú ròu] beef
牛蛙[niú wā] bullfrog

浓脓弄 NONG
浓 nóng
浓缩[nóng suō] concentration ~ 果汁 concentrated fruit juice/ ~ 丸 concentrated pills/ ~ 维生素 concentrated vitamin

脓 nóng
脓疮[nóng chuāng] running sore
脓耳[nóng ěr] suppurative otitis media
脓痂[nóng jiā] puric crust ~ 脱落，新

肌生起,病可痊愈。After exfoliation of the puric crust and regeneration of new tissues the illness is nearly cured.

脓疱 [nóng pào] pustule

脓痰 [nóng tán] purulent sputum 咳吐 ~ 不止 keeping on coughing out purulent sputum

脓血 [nóng xuè] purulent blood ~ 便 bloody purulent feces/ ~ 痢 dysentery with passing bloody purulent feces

脓肿 [nóng zhǒng] abscess 肺 ~ pulmonary abscess

弄 nòng

弄舌 [nòng shé] tongue waggling ~ 多由心脾积热引起。Tongue waggling is mainly due to accumulated heat in the heart and spleen.

衄怒 NU

衄 nǔ

衄肉攀睛 [nǔ ròu pān jīng] pterygium

怒 nù

怒 [nù] anger ~ 伤肝 liver impaired by rage/ ~ 则气上。Rage drives qi upward.

女衄 Nü

女 nǔ

女科 [nǔ kē] (department of) gynecology and obstetrics ~ 病 women's diseases

女劳复 [nǔ láo fù] sexual taxation relapse

女子胞 [nǔ zǐ bāo] uterus, womb ~ 为奇恒之府之一。The uterus is one of the extraordinary organs.

衄 nù

衄家 [nù jiā] patient with frequent epistaxis ~ 不可发汗,因为血汗同源。In treatment for frequent epistaxis the sweating method cannot be used, because sweat and blood are of the same source.

衄血 [nù xuè] epistaxis

暖 NUAN

暖 nuǎn

暖背 [nuǎn bèi] keeping the back warm

暖宫 [nuǎn gōng] warming the uterus ~ 祛瘀 warming the uterus and eliminating blood stasis

暖脾胃 [nuǎn pí wèi] warming the spleen and stomach 补肝肾, ~ reinforcing the liver and kidney, warming the spleen and stomach/ ~ 法多用于治疗脾胃虚寒证。Warming the spleen and stomach is adopted for a deficiency pattern of the spleen and stomach.

暖气 [nuǎn qì] central heating

暖肾 [nuǎn shèn] warming the kidney ~ 温中 warming the kidney and middle-energizer/ ~ 法,多用于治疗肾阳虚证。For the pattern of deficiency of kidney-yang the method of warming the kidney is employed.

疟 NUE

疟 nüè

疟疾［nüè ji］malaria

O

呕偶藕 OU

呕 ǒu

呕家［ǒu jiā］habitual vomiter ～不可甘。It is forbidden to give sweet stuffs for habitual vomiters.

呕逆［ǒu nì］vomiting

呕乳［ǒu rǔ］milk vomiting

呕吐［ǒu tù］vomiting ～清涎 vomiting clear mucus/～宿食 vomiting retained food/～酸腐 vomiting sour fetid matter

呕血［ǒu xuè］hematemesis

偶 ǒu

偶刺［ǒu cì］paired needling ～疗法 paired needling therapy

偶方［ǒu fāng］formulas with ingredients even in number

藕 ǒu

藕粉［ǒu fěn］lotus root starch 冲～。Prepare some lotus root paste.

P

拍排 PAI

拍 pāi

拍法［pāi fǎ］patting ～以手腕发力,平稳而有节奏地拍打患部。Patting is applied by using the wrist strength to tap the affected part rhythmically.

排 pái

排除杂念［pái chú zá niàn］ridding distraction ～,集中注意力。Rid distraction and focus your attention.

排毒［pái dú］driving toxic substances out ～养颜 driving toxic substances out to preserve one's fine complexion

排骨［pái gǔ］spare rib ～汤 pork rib soup/红烧～ pork ribs braised in soy sauce

排罐法［pái guàn fǎ］multiple cupping in alignment 采用 ~ aligning a number of cups on the affected area

排脓［pái nóng］evacuating pus ~ 托毒 evacuating pus and toxic substances

排针［pái zhēn］withdrawal of a needle

盘 PAN
盘 pán

盘香［pán xiāng］incense coil 点燃 ~ 常见于寺院道观或祠堂。The incense coil is usually burnt in Buddhist, Taoist or ancestral temples.

盘坐［pán zuò］sitting cross-legged 闭目 ~ sitting upright with the legs crossed and eyes closed/单 ~ single cross-legged sitting/双 ~ double cross-legged sitting

膀胖 PANG
膀 páng

膀胱经［páng guāng jīng］Urinary Bladder Meridian

膀胱湿热［páng guāng shī rè］dampness-heat in the urinary bladder

膀胱失约［páng guāng shī yuē］dysfunction of the urinary bladder

胖 pàng

胖大舌［pàng dà shé］enlarged tongue

胖头鱼［pàng tóu yú］big-head carp

炮泡疱 PAO
炮 páo

炮制［páo zhì］processing ~ 工艺 processing techniques/ ~ 方法 processing methods/ ~原则 processing principles/从古至今，中药的 ~ 方法也有所演变和发展。Throughout history methods of processing herbs have evolved and developed. / ~ 可以加强草药疗效或去除毒性。Herbal processing can strengthen efficacy or remove poisonous substances.

泡 pào

泡［pào］soaking ~ 药 bathing herbal medicinals/ ~ 服 taken in the form of a decoction/ ~ 腾片 effervescent tablet

疱 pào

疱疹［pào zhěn］herpes 单纯 ~ herpes simplex/带状 ~ herpes zoster/带状 ~ 是常见的皮肤科疾病。Herps zoster is a commonly-seen skin disease.

培配 PEI
培 péi

培土［péi tǔ］building up earth phase（spleen）~ 生金 building up earth phase（spleen）to generate metal phase（lung）/ ~ 抑木 building up earth phase（spleen）to restrict wood phase（liver）

配 pèi

配方［pèi fāng］making a prescription 饮食 ~ food recipe

配伍［pèi wǔ］combination of the herbal ingredients ~ 恰当 proper combination of the herbal ingredients/药物经过适

当的 ~ 后能增强疗效。Combination of herbal ingredients can strengthen the efficacy.

配穴 [pèi xué] auxiliary acupoint selected ~ 处方 prescription of auxiliary acupoints/根据疾病的性质选穴 ~。Select the main acupoints and the auxiliary ones according to the nature of a disease.

配药[pèi yào] filling a prescription

配制 [pèi zhì] preparing ~ 成丸剂 preparing the ingredients into pills

喷盆 PEN

喷 pēn

喷嚏[pēn tì] sneezing

盆 pén

盆菜[pén cài] ready-to-cook dish

烹 PENG

烹 pēng

烹茶[pēng chá] making tea

烹饪 [pēng rèn] cooking ~ 比赛 cooking competition/ ~ 法 cookery/ ~ 技艺 cooking skills/学习 ~ 技艺 learning cooking skills

烹调 [pēng tiáo] cooking ~ 技术 cooking skills 我妈的 ~ 手艺很好。My mother is quite a cook.

劈皮疲琵脾痞劈僻 PI

劈 pī

劈法[pī fǎ] striking with the ulnar side of the palm

皮 pí

皮痹[pí bì] painful and numb skin

皮部[pí bù] cutaneous region ~ 是经脉支配的局部体表皮肤。The cutaneous region refers to the topical superficial skin dominated by meridians.

皮刺 [pí cì] skin needling 沿 ~ puncturing along the skin surface

皮肤粗糙[pí fū cū cāo] rough skin 热病伤阴, 肌肤失养, ~。A febrile disease impairs yin, leading to rough skin due to malnutrition of the skin and muscles.

皮肤干燥[pí fū gān zào] dry skin

皮肤老化[pí fū lǎo huà] skin ageing 阳光暴晒, 易使 ~。Exposure to the blazing sun is easy to cause skin ageing.

皮肤宜常干沐[pí fū yí cháng gān mù] frequent dry-clean of the skin ~ 有助于气血流通。Frequent dry-clean of the skin helps smooth circulation of qi and blood.

皮肤针[pí fū zhēn] dermal needling ~ 疗法 dermal needling therapy

皮内针 [pí nèi zhēn] intradermal needling

皮水[pí shuǐ] general edema

皮屑[pí xiè] scurf 头 ~ dandruff

皮针[pí zhēn] sword-shaped needle ~ 疗法 sword-shaped needling therapy

疲 pí

疲乏[pí fá] tired

疲劳极限［pí láo jí xiàn］endurance limit

琵 pí

琵琶［pí pa］*pipa*（Chinese stringed musical instrument with a fretted fingerboard）

脾 pí

脾［pí］spleen ~ 主口 The condition of the mouth reflects the condition of the spleen.

脾病忌酸［pí bìng jì suān］sour flavor abstained in patients with spleen disorders

脾不统血［pí bù tǒng xuè］failure of the spleen to control blood vessels

脾藏意［pí cáng yì］idea housed in the spleen

脾藏营［pí cáng yíng］nutrients stored in the spleen

脾经［pí jīng］Spleen Meridian

脾开窍于口［pí kāi qiào yú kǒu］mouth, the window of the spleen

脾气健运［pí qì jiàn yùn］normal functioning of the spleen in transportation

脾失健运［pí shī jiàn yùn］dysfunction of the spleen in transportation

脾胃［pí wèi］spleen and stomach ~ 不和 disharmony between the spleen and stomach/ ~ 湿热 dampness-heat in the spleen and stomach/ ~ 阳虚 yang deficiency of the spleen and stomach/ 内伤 ~，百病由生。All diseases arise from injury to the spleen and stomach.

脾为后天之本［pí wéi hòu tiān zhī běn］spleen, the root of the human acquired ability

脾为生痰之源［pí wéi shēng tán zhī yuán］spleen, the source of sputum

脾泄［pí xiè］diarrhea due to deficiency in the spleen

脾约［pí yuē］constipation due to dysfunction of the spleen

脾主肌肉［pí zhǔ jī ròu］muscles dominated by the spleen

脾主运化［pí zhǔ yùn huà］transportation and transformation governed by the spleen

痞 pǐ

痞满［pǐ mǎn］stuffiness and fullness

劈 pǐ

劈叉［pǐ chà］doing the splits

僻 pì

僻邪［pì xié］pathogenic factors ~ 不至,长生久视。If one can avoid the attack by pathogenic factors, he will be able to live a long life.

偏片 PIAN

偏 piān

偏差［piān chā］deviation

偏方［piān fāng］special but irregular recipe 搜集 ~ collecting special but irregular recipes. / ~ 有时可以收到明显的疗效。Special but irregular recipes can sometimes bring a significant effect.

P

偏食［piān shí］preference for some food 虫证可见 ~ 。Special liking for some stuff is a common sign in parasite-induced disorders. /若 ~ 肉类, 少食蔬菜, 容易致病。Eating more meat and fewer vegetables may lead to disease.

偏瘫［piān tān］hemiplegia

偏头痛［piān tóu tòng］migraine

片 piàn

片儿汤［piàn ér tāng］soup with flat pieces of dough cooked in it

片剂［piàn jì］tablet

漂 PIAO
漂 piǎo

漂药［piǎo yào］rinsing medicinal herbs ~ 能够清除药材表面的尘垢。After the medicinal herbs are rinsed, the superficial dirt is removed.

频品 PIN
频 pín

频服［pín fú］frequently taken in small dose 催吐药应 ~ 。Herbal emetics should be given in small portions at intervals.

品 pǐn

品尝［pǐn cháng］tasting

品茗［pǐn míng］sipping tea（to judge its quality）

品香［pǐn xiāng］smelling incense smoke 放松心情 ~ 。Smell the incense smoke with a peaceful mind.

平 PING
平 píng

平补法［píng bǔ fǎ］moderate reinforcement

平补平泻［píng bǔ píng xiè］moderate reinforcing-reducing method 目前多以中等的捻转、提插为 ~ 。At present, the moderate reinforcing and reducing method means neither strong nor light force is used in twirling, lifting and thrusting needles in acupuncture.

平旦［píng dàn］dawn ~ 服 medicinals taken before breakfast/ ~ 人气生 Yang-qi in the body starts to rise in the morning.

平肝潜阳［píng gān qián yáng］pacifying the liver and subduing yang

平和质［píng hé zhì］type of balanced constitution

平衡膳食［píng héng shàn shí］balanced diet ~ 是当今饮食的生活指南。Currently balanced diet is the guide to life. / ~ 是防止原发性高血压的基石。Balanced diet is the cornerstone to prevent primary hypertension. / ~ 与人体健康密切相关。Balanced diet is closely related to human health.

平人［píng rén］healthy person ~ 之脉 healthy person's pulse/ ~ 不食饮七日而死者,小谷精气津液皆尽故也。

Healthy people may die without taking food and drinking water for 7 days because of complete exhaustion of food essence and body fluids. / ~ 而气胜形者寿。 A healthy person who has abundant qi but seems not strong may enjoy a long life. / ~ 之脉富有胃气。 Healthy person's pulse is always full of stomach-qi.

平卧[píng wò] lying flat

平息[píng xī] normal breathing

平治于权衡[píng zhì yú quán héng] keeping balance of yin and yang

破魄 PO
破 pò

破血[pò xuè] removing blood stasis with drastic medicinals

破阳[pò yáng] first sexual intercourse for boys 男子 ~ 太早, 则伤精气。 Essence is impaired in boys who have sexual intercourse too early.

破阴[pò yīn] first sexual intercourse for girls 女子 ~ 太早, 则伤血脉。 Blood is impaired in girls who have first sexual intercourse too early.

魄 pò

魄[pò] corporeal soul 肺藏 ~ corporeal soul stored in the lung

扑 PU
扑 pū

扑粉[pū fěn] applying medicinal powder

Q

七齐奇脐歧崎棋起气器 QI
七 qī

七冲门[qī chōng mén] seven important portals

七方[qī fāng] seven formulas 制方之用, 大、小、缓、急、奇、偶、复 ~ 是也。 The seven formulas refer to the major, minor, slow-acting, quick-acing and compound formulas together with formulas with ingredients odd and even in number.

七窍[qī qiào] seven orifices of the human head ~ 流血 bleeding from one's mouth, nostrils, eyes and ears

七情[qī qíng] seven emotions ~ 六欲 various emotions and desires/病之内生者, 生于 ~ 过极。 Diseases may occur as a result of seven emotional stress.

七伤[qī shāng] seven kinds of impairment 五劳、六极 ~ 多致虚劳。

Q

Five kinds of strain, six kinds of exhaustion and seven kinds of impairment may cause consumptive disease.

七损八益[qī sǔn bā yì] seven ills and eight benefits ~ 乃房中要诀。The seven ills and eight benefits are the knack in sexual life.

七曜[qī yào] seven stars ~ 纬虚,五行丽地。The seven stars are orbiting in the sky and the five phases are affiliated to the earth. ~ 周旋 The seven stars are circling round in the sky.

齐 qí

齐刺[qí cì] triple needling

奇 qí

奇恒之腑[qí héng zhī fǔ] extraordinary organs

奇经八脉[qí jīng bā mài] eight extra meridians ~ 是经络系统的重要组成部分。The eight extra meridians are the important component part of the meridian system.

奇邪[qí xié] unusual pathogenic factor

奇穴[qí xué] extra acupoint

脐 qí

脐风[qí fēng] tetanus

歧 qí

歧骨[qí gǔ] bone juncture

崎 qí

崎岖[qí qū] rugged 山路 ~ rugged mountain path/ ~ 坎坷的人生道路 rough and rugged paths of life

棋 qí

棋艺[qí yì] chess skill ~ 精湛 being a chess expert/他们俩在切磋 ~。They are playing chess and want to see what they can learn from each other.

棋友[qí yǒu] chess friend

起 qǐ

起罐[qǐ guàn] cup removal

起居[qǐ jū] daily life ~ 不节 living an irregular life / ~ 有常 leading a regular life / ~ 有常,延年益寿 Leading a regular life ensures long life./她妈妈 ~ 饮食都很规律,所以长寿。Her mother keeps a strict regimen in all aspects of her daily life, so she has enjoyed a long life.

起卧有时[qǐ wò yǒu shí] rising and going to bed at regular time ~ 是长寿老人的共同特点。Many long lived senior citizens share a common character of getting up and sleeping in regular hours.

起针[qǐ zhēn] withdrawal of a needle 急 ~ quick withdrawal of a needle/慢 ~ slow withdrawal of a needle

气 qì

气[qì] qi, chee, chi ~ 闭 obstruction of qi/ ~ 常有余,血常不足。Qi is often surplus and blood is often scanty. / ~ 之在人, 和则为正气,不和则为邪气。Qi moving normally in the body is known as healthy qi, while qi moving abnormally is called the pathogenic factor. /百病皆生于～。 All diseases result from qi disorder. /人以天地之～生, 四时之法成。 Human beings come into existence as the result of the qi of the Heaven and Earth in accordance with the laws of the four seasons.

气闭[qì bì] obstruction of qi

气布而蕃育 [qì bù ér fán yù] reproduction based on qi laying out

气喘 [qì chuǎn] panting 咳嗽～ coughing and panting ～不得卧 failure to lie flat due to panting

气粗声高[qì cū shēng gāo] harsh breathing and sonorous sound

气促[qì cù] shortness of breath

气大伤人 [qì dà shāng rén] health injured by raving anger

气的升降出入[qì de shēng jiàng chū rù] ascending, descending, exiting and entering of qi

气短[qì duǎn] shortness of breath

气分[qì fēn] qi level 热入～ invasion of the qi level by heat/～大热, 口大渴, 汗大出, 脉洪大, 白虎汤主之。 Excessive heat in the qi level manifested itself as a high fever, extreme thirst, profuse sweating and full pulse, for which the *Baihu* Decoction is the first choice.

气刚者 [qì gāng zhě] strong-willed person

气功[qì gōng] *qigong* ～疗法 *qigong* therapy/道家 ～ Taoist *qigong*/佛家 ～ Buddhist *qigong*/健身 ～ *qigong* for keeping fit/儒家 ～ Confucian *qigong*/武术 ～ martial-art *qigong*/医学 ～ medical *qigong*

气功偏差[qì gōng piān chā] adverse reaction in *qigong*

气臌[qì gǔ] tympanites

气候[qì hòu] climate

气化[qì huà] transformation of qi ～不利 disturbance in qi transformation/～无权 failure of qi transformation/胃之 ～失职小便不利。 Difficulty of urination arises from failure of well functioning of stomach-qi.

气会膻中 [qì huì dàn zhōng] qi assembling at Danzhong (CV 17) ～, 故治疗气病多选此穴。Danzhong (CV 17) is usually selected in treatment for qi-related disorders since qi assembles here.

气机[qì jī] qi activity ～不利 disorder of qi activity/～郁滞 impeded qi activity

气街[qì jiē] qi path

气口[qì kǒu] wrist pulse ～诊法 wrist pulse-taking method

气满者 [qì mǎn zhě] person with stagnated qi ～, 不思食。 A person with stagnated qi often has poor appetite.

Q

气门[qì mén] sweat pore

气逆[qì nì] adverse rising of qi 怒则~。Qi flows upward when angry.

气强者[qì qiáng zhě] high and mighty person

气清者[qì qīng zhě] clear-headed person ~聪明贤达 A clear-headed person is usually full of talent and wisdom.

气柔者[qì róu zhě] person with tenderness ~慈仁淳笃 A person with tenderness is benevolent and honest.

气色[qì sè] complexion 近来你的~不好。You have not been looking well recently.

气始而生化[qì shǐ ér shēng huà] production and transformation based on formation of qi

气随血脱[qì suí xuè tuō] loss of blood leading to qi collapse

气脱[qì tuō] qi collapse

气为血帅[qì wéi xuè shuài] qi, the commander of blood ~,血为气母。Qi is the commander of blood and blood (is) the mother of qi.

气陷[qì xiàn] sinking of qi

气行[qì xíng] smooth flow of qi 勇者~则已,怯者则着而为病也。One with a strong physique has smooth flow of qi. On the contrary, one may fall ill owing to impeded flow of qi.

气胸[qì xiōng] pneumothorax

气虚[qì xū] qi deficiency ~发热 fever in qi deficiency/ ~则寒,血虚则热。Cold is caused by qi deficiency, whereas heat by deficiency of blood.

气虚质[qì xū zhì] type of qi-deficiency constitution ~需益气健脾。For people with the qi-deficiency constitution it is advisable to reinforce qi and invigorate the spleen.

气血[qì xuè] qi and blood ~畅通 smooth circulation of qi and blood/ ~通调 regulating qi and blood flow/ ~两燔 excessive heat in both qi and blood levels/ ~两虚 deficiency of both qi and blood/ ~正平 harmony between qi and blood/营卫相谐, ~畅通,人自安和。One is healthy as long as the nutritive and defensive levels are in harmony and qi and blood in smooth circulation. / ~上荣,耳聪目明。Good eyes and ears depend on the head nourished by qi and blood.

气郁质[qì yù zhì] type of qi-stagnation constitution ~需疏肝理气。For people with the qi-stagnation constitution it is advisable to promote circulation of liver-qi.

气胀[qì zhàng] abdominal distension and fullness due to frustration

气质[qì zhì] temperament; quality 良好~fine quality

气滞[qì zhì] stagnation of qi ~腹痛 abdominal pain with qi stagnation/ ~血瘀 qi stagnation with blood stasis/ ~腰痛,不得俯仰。Lower back pain due to qi stagnation makes one difficult to bend forward and backward.

气肿［qì zhǒng］edema due to disorder of qi

器 qì

器质［qì zhì］structure（of the human organs）~性疾病 organic disease

牵谦前潜浅 QIAN

牵 qiān

牵拉法［qiān lā fǎ］traction

牵引［qiān yǐn］traction 骨骼 ~ skeletal traction/颈 ~ cervical traction/ ~ 推拿法 traction with *tuina*-massage maneuvers

谦 qiān

谦和［qiān hé］modest and kind 态度 ~ modest and amiable attitude

谦受益［qiān shòu yì］modesty being beneficial ~, 满招损。Modesty is beneficial and conceit detrimental.

前 qián

前后配穴法［qián hòu pèi xué fǎ］front and back acupoint combination ~ 用于脏腑同病。The front and back acupoint combination is applied to treating disorders of the *zang-fu* organs.

前后正中线［qián hòu zhèng zhōng xiàn］anterior-posterior midline

前阴［qián yīn］external genitals

潜 qián

潜能［qián néng］potential 发掘 ~ drawing out one's potentials

潜心淡意［qián xīn dàn yì］concentration on something with fewer desires ~, 不使邪念妄生, 是节欲的关键。Concentration on something with fewer desires keeps away evil intention, and it is the key to continence.

潜阳安神［qián yáng ān shén］subduing hyperactivity of liver-yang to calm the mind ~ 对治疗失眠有良好疗效。Insomnia responds well to subduing liver-yang to calm the mind.

潜镇［qián zhèn］subduing hyperactivity and tranquilizing ~ 肝阳 subduing hyperactivity of liver-yang and tranquilizing

浅 qiǎn

浅刺［qiǎn cì］shallow needling ~ 拔罐法 shallow needling with cupping/额部、脚部穴位应 ~。The shallow needling is applied to the acupoints located at the forehead and foot.

强 QIANG

强 qiáng

强刺激［qiáng cì jī］strong stimulation 体虚之人宜 ~, 以利其气。Strong stimulation is given to debilitated patients to get the acupuncture sensation soon.

强筋健骨［qiáng jīn jiàn gǔ］toning up

muscles and bones 经常锻炼身体可以 ~ 。Regular exercise tones up muscles and bones.

强人[qiáng rén] strong tall man ~ 服药, 可增大一定的剂量。A higher dosage of medicine is given to a strong and tall man.

强项[qiáng xiàng] strong point

强腰脊[qiáng yāo jǐ] toning up the spinal column

强壮[qiáng zhuàng] strong ~ 功 fitness qigong 这补药能 ~ 病人体质。The tonic can build up a patient's physique.

切切怯 QIE
切 qiē

切法[qiē fǎ] pressing method ~ 可以在进针时减轻疼痛, 促使得气。The pressing method helps ease pain on insertion of a needle and induce qi arrival.

切 qiè

切脉[qiè mài] pulse-taking ~ 是中医四种诊法之一。Pulse-taking is one of the four diagnostic examinations in traditional Chinese medicine.

切诊[qiè zhěn] pulse-taking and palpation

怯 qiè

怯人[qiè rén] coward ~ 胆气虚。A coward usually suffers from deficiency of gallbladder-qi.

琴勤噙寝揿 QIN
琴 qín

琴棋书画[qín qí shū huà] music, chess, calligraphy and painting ~ 能陶冶情操。Music, chess, calligraphy and painting shape one's values. / ~ 养生 using music, chess, calligraphy and painting to build up health

琴瑟[qín sè] marital harmony ~ 不调 discord between husband and wife

勤 qín

勤求古训, 博采众长[qín qiú gǔ xùn, bó cǎi zhòng cháng] seeking ancient maxim industriously, discovering and making use of the strong points of all others

噙 qín

噙化[qín huà] sucking

寝 qǐn

寝不语[qǐn bù yǔ] not talking when going to sleep ~ 可以防止失眠。Do not talk when one is going to sleep, which is a way to prevent sleeplessness.

寝汗[qǐn hàn] sweating in sleep due to weakness ~ 出憎风 night sweating with aversion to wind

揿 qìn

揿针[qìn zhēn] thumbtack needle ~ 体形小, 运用于皮下埋藏。Small in size, the thumbtack needle is applicable to subcutaneous embedding.

青轻清情 QING

青 qīng

青带［qīng dài］leukorrhagia with greenish discharge ~多湿。Excessive dampness contributes to leukorrhagia with greenish discharge.

青风内障［qīng fēng nèi zhàng］simple glaucoma

青山绿水［qīng shān lǜ shuǐ］blue mountains and green waters ~赏心悦目，令人陶醉。Blue mountains and green waters delight both the eyes and the mind, and people are enchanted.

青紫［qīng zǐ］cynosis ~舌 bluish-purple tongue

轻 qīng

轻剂［qīng jì］mild diaphoretic formula ~通常用来治疗轻浅在表的疾病。Mild diaphoretic formulas are usually adopted in treatment for mild conditions.

轻取［qīng qǔ］taking pulse gently

轻身［qīng shēn］light body; weight loss

轻松［qīng sōng］relaxed; lighthearted 心情 ~with a lightsome heart

轻下［qīng xià］mild purgation

轻症［qīng zhèng］mild case 新冠 ~mild case of COVID-19

清 qīng

清便自调［qīng biàn zì tiáo］normal bowel movement

清炒［qīng chǎo］sole stir-frying 某些药物炮制法为 ~ Sole stir-frying is used in processing some herbal medicinals.

清淡［qīng dàn］light ~食物 light food

清炖［qīng dùn］boiling in clear soup without soy sauce ~鸭 stewed duck without soy sauce

清法［qīng fǎ］heat clearing ~用于治疗热证。The heat-clearing method is applied to a heat pattern.

清化痰热［qīng huà tán rè］clearing heat and phlegm 黄芩具有 ~之效。*Huangqin*（Baical Skullcap Root）acts to clear heat and phlegm.

清解胎毒［qīng jiě tāi dú］eliminating fetal virulence ~属于中医清解之法。Eliminating fetal virulence is a heat clearance method in traditional Chinese medicine.

清静无为［qīng jìng wú wéi］being quiet and having fewer desires 老子崇尚自然，主张 ~。Laozi advocated nature and held "being quiet and having fewer desires". / ~以养神存身，治病于未然。Discard all desires and worries from one's mind to keep fit and put prevention first.

清冷［qīng lěng］chilly ~的夜晚 chilly night

清里泻热［qīng lǐ xiè rè］clearing internal heat 白虎汤可以 ~。The *Baihu* Decoction acts to clear internal heat.

清明[qīng míng] pure brightness

清明节[qīng míng jié] Tomb Sweeping Day

清气分热[qīng qì fèn rè] clearing heat from the qi level ~ 的方剂,具有清热除烦,生津止咳的作用。Formulas for clearing heat from the qi level act to remove heat, eliminate vexation and promote the generation of fluid to quench thirst.

清气凉营[qīng qì liáng yíng] removing heat from the qi and nutritive levels ~ 适用于温热病气营两燔。The therapeutic method of removing heat from the qi and nutritive levels is applicable to intense heat in the qi and nutritive levels in warm-heat diseases.

清热[qīng rè] clearing heat ~ 剂 formulas that clear heat

清热化痰[qīng rè huà tán] clearing heat and resolving phlegm

清热解表[qīng rè jiě biǎo] clearing heat and releasing the exterior

清热解毒[qīng rè jiě dú] clearing heat and toxic substances

清热解暑[qīng rè jiě shǔ] clearing summer-heat ~ 类药多在夏季使用。Medicinals acting to clear summer-heat are mainly prescribed in summer.

清热开窍[qīng rè kāi qiào] clearing heat to resuscitate

清热燥湿[qīng rè zào shī] removing heat and dampness

清透郁热[qīng tòu yù rè] removing stagnated heat

清心[qīng xīn] clearing heart-fire; getting rid of distracting thoughts ~ 安神 clearing heart-fire to calm the mind/ ~ 开窍 clearing heart-fire to regain consciousness

清心寡欲[qīng xīn guǎ yù] being pure of the heart and having fewer desires

清心火[qīng xīn huǒ] clearing heart-fire ~ 、养心阴、安心神。Clear heart-fire, replenish heart-yin and tranquilize the mind

清虚静泰[qīng xū jìng tài] sober with a stable mind

清虚热[qīng xū rè] clearing heat in a deficiency condition

清阳[qīng yáng] lucid yang-qi ~ 不升 failure of lucid yang-qi to rise/ ~ 出上窍, 浊阴出下窍。Lucid yang (usable substance) ascends to the upper orifices, and turbid yin (unusable substance) descends to the lower orifices.

清营凉血[qīng yíng liáng xuè] clearing heat from the nutritive and blood levels

清脏腑热[qīng zàng fǔ rè] clearing heat from the zang-fu organs ~ 法适用于各类里热证。Clearing heat from the zang-fu organs is applicable to various internal heat patterns.

清蒸[qīng zhēng] steaming in clear

soup without soy sauce ~鱼 steamed fish

情 qíng

情意[qíng yì] affection 友好 ~ friendly sentiment

情欲[qíng yù] lust ~ 适度 moderating sentiment and desire

情志[qíng zhì] moods; emotions ~ 不畅 moodiness/~ 过极 heightened emotional sensitivity/~ 互胜 the inter-restriction relationship between emotions/调摄 ~ adjusting emotions/~ 中和 even-handed emotions/养生应重视调节 ~。Attention should be paid to regulation of sentiment in health preservation.

秋 QIU

秋 qiū

秋冬养阴[qiū dōng yǎng yīn] replenishing yin in autumn and winter

秋分[qiū fēn] Autumn Equinox

秋季养生[qiū jì yǎng shēng] health preservation in autumn

秋毛[qiū máo] weak and floating pulse seen in autumn

秋燥[qiū zào] autumn dryness ~ 伤肺 Autumn dryness often impairs the lung.

驱祛趋取龋去趣 QU

驱 qū

驱虫[qū chóng] expelling intestinal parasites ~药 anthelmintics

祛 qū

祛风[qū fēng] expelling wind ~ 活血 expelling wind and activating blood circulation/防风是 ~ 良药，既可祛外风，也可祛内风。*Fangfeng* (Divaricate Saposhnikovia Root) is a good remedy which acts not only to expel external but also internal wind.

祛风除湿[qū fēng chú shī] expelling wind-dampness ~ 止痛。Pain is relieved by way of expelling wind-dampness.

祛风定惊[qū fēng dìng jīng] expelling wind to relieve convulsion ~ 常用治小儿热极生风所致的惊厥证。Expelling wind to relieve convulsion is often adopted to treat infantile convulsion caused by intense heat.

祛风解表[qū fēng jiě biǎo] expelling wind to release the exterior 荆芥具有 ~ 之功效 *Jingjie* (Fineleaf Schizonepeta Herb) acts to release an exterior pattern by expelling wind.

祛寒湿[qū hán shī] expelling cold-dampness 寒痹者宜温阳 ~、止痛利关节。It is essential to invigorate yang and expel cold-dampness to treat impediment due to cold to relieve pain and thus achieve free movement of joints.

祛痰[qū tán] eliminating phlegm ~ 开窍 eliminating phlegm to regain consciousness

Q

祛邪［qū xié］eliminating pathogenic factors ~ 扶正 eliminating pathogenic factors to restore healthy qi

祛瘀［qū yū］eliminating blood stasis ~ 活血 eliminating blood stasis to activate blood circulation/ ~ 生新 eliminating blood stasis to induce regeneration of tissues/ ~ 消肿 eliminating blood stasis to subside a swelling

趋 qū

趋利避害［qū lì bì hài］seeking advantages and avoiding disadvantages

取 qǔ

取穴法［qǔ xué fǎ］acupoint selection principle

龋 qǔ

龋齿［qǔ chǐ］dental caries 预防 ~ prevention of dental caries/儿童多食甘味,易致 ~。Children are apt to have dental caries because they prefer sweet food.

去 qù

去陈［qù chén］eliminating staleness and stagnation ~ 有改善人体内循环的作用。Eliminating staleness and stagnation may improve the internal recycle.

去腐［qù fǔ］removing necrotic tissue ~ 生肌 removing necrotic tissues and promote regeneration of new tissues.

去火毒［qù huǒ dú］removing toxic fire

去欲［qù yù］discarding desires 老子之 ~ 包含两个方面。Discarding desires has two meanings according to Laozi.

趣 qù

趣味［qù wèi］fun, taste ~ 盎然 full of interest/ ~ 高雅 good taste/ ~ 索然 poor taste

全拳 QUAN

全 quán

全才［quán cái］all-rounder

全面膳食［quán miàn shàn shí］all-round diet ~ ,平衡膳食都是现代营养学所提倡的。All-round and balanced diet is advocated by modern nutriology.

全身浮肿［quán shēn fú zhǒng］general dropsy ~ 责之于脾胃虚弱。General dropsy lays blame on weakness of the spleen and stomach.

全身痛［quán shēn tòng］general pain

全身无力［quán shēn wú lì］general weakness 大病后,气血俱虚,~。Patients may have general weakness from a serious disease as their qi and blood are in a deficient state.

拳 quán

拳术［quán shù］Chinese boxing

缺却雀 QUE

缺 quē

缺乳［quē rǔ］lack of lactation

却 què

却谷食气［què gǔ shí qì］qi feeding

instead of food feeding

却老[què lǎo] delaying senescence

雀 què

雀斑[què bān] freckle

雀目[què mù] night blindness

雀啄灸［què zhuó jiǔ］bird-pecking moxibustion

雀啄脉［què zhuó mài］bird-pecking pulse ~ 主脾胃之气已绝。Bird-pecking pulse suggests exhaustion of the qi of the spleen and stomach.

R

染 RAN

染 rǎn

染苔[rǎn tāi] stained tongue coating

桡 RAO

桡 ráo

桡骨[ráo gǔ] radius ~ 骨折 fracture of the radius

热 RE

热 rè

热病[rè bìng] febrile disease, fever ~ 少愈, 食肉则复 When one has a fever or the fever slightly subsides, eating meat may cause a relapse.

热不炙唇[rè bù zhì chún] hot food that does not scald lips ~, 冷不振齿 hot food that does not scald lips, and cold food that does not chill teeth

热毒[rè dú] toxic heat ~ 闭肺 toxic heat plugged in the lung/ ~ 痢 toxic-heat dysentery/ ~疥疮 toxic-heat sore

热敷[rè fū] hot medicated compress

热服[rè fú] decoction taken hot 某些汤药 ~, 效果更好。Some herbal decoctions are more effective if taken hot.

热伏冲任［rè fú chōng rèn］heat lodging in the Thoroughfare Vessel and Conception Vessel

热极生风［rè jí shēng fēng］intense heat generating wind

热极生寒［rè jí shēng hán］cold generated by intense heat

热结[rè jié] heat retention ~膀胱 heat retained in the urinary bladder

热淋[rè lìn] stranguria due to heat

热情［rè qíng］enthusiasm ~ 款待 treating cordially

热入心包［rè rù xīn bāo］invasion of the pericardium by heat

热入血室[rè rù xuè shì] invasion of the uterus by heat

热伤津液[rè shāng jīn yè] body fluid consumed by heat

热伤神明[rè shāng shén míng] heat disturbing mental activities

热盛[rè shèng] intense heat ~则肿 swelling due to intense heat

热手擦面[rè shǒu cā miàn] rubbing the face with warm hands ~可改善面部血液循环。Rubbing the face with warm hands can improve facial blood circulation.

热水浴[rè shuǐ yù] hot water bath ~时间不宜过长。Never take a long-time hot water bath.

热无犯热[rè wú fàn rè] non-administration of remedies hot in property in summer without cold manifestations

热性[rè xìng] hot property of medicinals

热药[rè yào] hot-property medicinals ~伤阴 Hot-property medicinals impair yin. /寒证用~。Hot-property medicinals are effective for a cold pattern.

R

热因热用[rè yīn rè yòng] using medicinals warm or hot in property for pseudo-heat symptoms

热者寒之[rè zhě hán zhī] medicinals cold in property prescribed for a heat pattern ~,寒者热之。A heat pattern is relieved with cold-property medicinals, while a cold pattern is relieved with hot-property medicinals.

热证[rè zhèng] heat pattern

人仁忍任妊 REN

人 rén

人背复位[rén bèi fù wèi] back-carrying reduction

人痘接种[rén dòu jiē zhòng] ancient oriental variolation ~可用于预防天花。The ancient oriental variolation was used to prevent smallpox.

人文景观[rén wén jǐng guān] human landscape ~欣赏 enjoying human landscape/ ~是社会、艺术和历史的产物。The human landscape is the product of the society, arts and history.

人迎脉[rén yíng mài] common carotid artery

人之初性本善[rén zhī chū xìng běn shàn] All humans are inherently good.

人中疔[rén zhōng dīng] philtrum deep-rooted boil ~者,须防其走黄。It is essential to prevent a philtrum deep-rooted boil from being complicated by septicemia.

人走茶凉[rén zǒu chá liáng] out of sight, out of mind

仁 rén

仁爱[rén ài] kind-hearted ~之心 kind heart

仁者寿[rén zhě shòu] long life enjoyed by benevolent people 孔子养生理论的精髓是"~"。"Long life enjoyed by benevolent people" is the quintessence of Confucian health preserving theory.

忍 rěn

忍便不解[rěn biàn bù jiě] holding back bowel movement ~易使毒素被肠组织黏膜吸收,危害身体。Holding back bowel movement harms health because some of the toxic materials in the feces would be absorbed by the intestinal mucous memberane.

忍急[rěn jí] subduing irritable mood ~戒怒 subduing irritable mood and keeping away from anger/养肝气要~戒怒。When liver-qi is being reinforced, it is essential to subdue irritable mood and keep away from anger.

任 rèn

任脉[rèn mài] Conception Vessel ~病 disorder of the Conception Vessel/~为病,男子内结七疝,女子带下瘕聚。When the Conception Vessel is diseased, seven kinds of hernia in males and morbid leukorrhea and abdominal mass in females may occur./~者,阴脉之海。The Conception Vessel is the reservoir of the yin meridians.

任其自然[rèn qí zì rán] Let nature take its course.

妊 rèn

妊娠恶阻[rèn shēn è zǔ] morning sickness

妊娠药忌[rèn shēn yào jì] medicament abstinence during pregnancy ~不能

绝对化。Medicament abstinence during pregnancy should not be observed absolutely.

日 RI
日 rì

日晡发(潮)热[rì bū fā (cháo) rè] tidal fever in late afternoon

日出而作[rì chū ér zuò] starting to work at sunrise 古人~,日落而息。Ancient people started to work at sun rise and rested at sunset.

日光浴[rì guāng yù] sunbath 进行~时不可入睡,以防止过多紫外线造成伤害。Never go asleep when having sunbath because long exposure to ultraviolet radiation damages the skin.

日中[rì zhōng] noontide ~而阳气隆 Yang-qi in the body reaches its peak in the noontide.

荣容 RONG
荣 róng

荣发固发[róng fà gù fà] nourishing and securing hair 梳头有疏通气血~的作用。Frequent combing hair helps promote circulation of qi and blood to nourish and secure hair.

荣枯老嫩[róng kū lǎo nèn] lustrous, withered, tough and tender-soft quality of the tongue texture 根据舌质的~,可判断疾病的虚实。According to the lustrous, withered, tough and tender-soft quality of the tongue texture, a deficiency or excess pattern can be judged.

荣辱防惊[róng rǔ fáng jīng] keeping a calm state of mind whenever one has honour or disgrace

荣养五脏[róng yǎng wǔ zàng] nurturing the five *zang*-organs ~ 不仅要均衡食物的性、色、味,还要均衡阴阳。In nurturing the five *zang*-organs not only the nature, color and flavor of food are cared, but also the balance of yin and yang.

容 róng

容平[róng píng] calm and tranquil 秋三月,此谓~。During the three months of autumn, all things are calm and tranquil.

柔揉肉 ROU

柔 róu

柔软体操[róu ruǎn tǐ cāo] calisthenics

柔术[róu shù] jujitsu

揉 róu

揉肚脐[róu dù qí] kneading the navel

揉法[róu fǎ] kneading maneuver ~ 可以和气血。Kneading is effective for regulating qi and blood.

肉 ròu

肉[ròu] muscle; flesh ~ 脱 emaciation

肉包子[ròu bāo zi] steamed bun with stuffing of minced meat

肉刺[ròu cì] clavus

肉瘤[ròu liú] sarcoma

肉人[ròu rén] strong and muscular person ~ ,针法以深刺为主。For a strong and muscular person it is advisable to insert a needle deeply in acupuncture therapy.

肉痿[ròu wěi] soft and weak muscle ~ 肢废 muscular atrophy and limb inability

如茹濡乳入褥 RU

如 rú

如法炮制[rú fǎ páo zhì] processing of medicinal herbs by the prescribed method 治病处方切忌 ~ 。Never follow a fixed example in treatment for diseases and in writing out a prescription.

如临深渊[rú lín shēn yuān] as though on the edge of an abyss

茹 rú

茹毛饮血[rú máo yǐn xuè] living a primitive life

茹素[rú sù] being a vegetarian

濡 rú

濡脉[rú mài] soggy pulse

乳 rǔ

乳癌[rǔ ái] breast cancer

乳蛾[rǔ é] tonsilitis

乳房[rǔ fáng] breast, mamma ~ 胀痛 mammary distending pain/ ~ 胀痛多见于肝气郁滞的病人。Mammary distending pain is usually found in patients with stagnation of liver-qi.

乳鸽[rǔ gē] squab

乳疽[rǔ jū] mammary cellulitis

乳痨[rǔ láo] infantile malnutrition

乳癖[rǔ pǐ] hyperplasia of the mammary gland

乳泣[rǔ qì] spontaneous lactorrhea

乳食不节[rǔ shí bù jié] improper feeding to infants ~易致小儿脾胃受伤。Improper feeding to infants easily causes impairment of the spleen and stomach.

乳牙[rǔ yá] deciduous tooth ~期 milk tooth period/~晚出 delayed eruption of the deciduous tooth/~早出 premature eruption of the deciduous tooth

乳痈[rǔ yōng] acute mastitis

乳晕[rǔ yùn] mammary areola

乳汁[rǔ zhī] breast milk ~不足 hypogalactia/~溢 lactorrhea

入 rù

入定[rù dìng] meditation in sitting

入静[rù jìng] in a composed state of mind ~放松 entering a composed state of mind and relaxing

入味儿[rù wèi er] tasty 这鱼挺~。The fish is quite tasty.

褥 rù

褥疮[rù chuāng] bedsore 多发性~ multiple bedsore

软 RUAN
软 ruǎn

软膏[ruǎn gāo] ointment 红霉素~ erythromycin ointment

软骨[ruǎn gǔ] cartilage

软坚[ruǎn jiān] softening a hard mass ~散结 softening and disintegrating masses

软气功[ruǎn qì gōng] soft *qigong*

软食[ruǎn shí] soft diet 老年人应多食用~。The senior should take more soft diet rather than hard one.

软组织损伤[ruǎn zǔ zhī sǔn shāng] soft tissue injury

润 RUN
润 rùn

润肠通便[rùn cháng tōng biàn] moistening the intestine to relieve constipation 蜂蜜具有~之功效。Honey works to relieve constipation by moistening the intestines.

润肺化痰[rùn fèi huà tán] moistening the lung and resolving phlegm 沙参具有~之功。*Shashen* (Coastal Glehnia Root) works to moisten the lung and resolve phlegm.

润肺养阴[rùn fèi yǎng yīn] moistening the lung to preserve yin

润肺止咳[rùn fèi zhǐ ké] moistening the lung to stop coughing 肺阴虚证所致咳嗽,应采用~法。Coughing due to deficiency of lung-yin is dealt with by moistening the lung to stop coughing.

润肤抗皱[rùn fū kàng zhòu] moistening the face to counteract wrinkles

R

润滑剂［rùn huá jì］lubricant

润苔［rùn tāi］moist tongue coating

润燥［rùn zào］moistening ～化痰 moistening and resolving phlegm/养阴～replenishing yin and moistening

弱若 RUO

弱 ruò

弱脉［ruò mài］weak pulse

若 ruò

若春无秋［ruò chūn wú qiū］the condition that appears as if there were only spring and no autumn

若冬无夏［ruò dōng wú xià］the condition that appears as if there were only winter and no summer

S

腮塞 SAI

腮 sāi

腮［sāi］cheek ～腺炎 mumps

腮肿欣燃［sāi zhǒng xīn rán］mumps with a burning sensation ～多由于火毒内盛而致。Mumps with a burning sensation is usually provoked by excessive internal toxic fire.

塞 sāi

塞法［sāi fǎ］insertion method ～指将药末包在纱布里塞入鼻孔、阴道或直肠的一种疗法。The insertion method is a therapeutic approach involving inserting some medicinal powder packed in gauze into the nostril, vagina or rectum.

塞因塞用［sāi yīn sāi yòng］treating the obstructive pattern with tonics

三散散 SAN

三 sān

三宝［sān bǎo］three treasures, three essentials ～并重 laying equal stress on the three essentials/精、气、神谓之～。Essence, qi and spirit are regarded as the three treasures.

三部九候［sān bù jiǔ hòu］three portions and nine positions for pulse-taking

三法［sān fǎ］three therapeutic methods：diaphoresis, emesis and purgation

三伏贴［sān fú tiē］plasters applied to acupoints in hottest days in summer

三焦［sān jiāo］triple energizer ～辨证 pattern differentiation according to the theory of the triple energizer/ ～咳 cough due to disorder of the triple energizer/ ~ 虚寒 cold in the triple energizer in a deficiency condition

三焦经 [sān jiāo jīng] Triple Energizer Meridian

三戒 [sān jiè] three admonitions 君子有 ~ :少之时,血气未定,戒之在色;及其壮也,血气方刚,戒之在斗;及其老也,血气既衰,戒之在得。 There are three admonitions for a man. When young and unable to control the sap of youth, the admonition for him is to guard against lust; when grown up to the prime of life and at his most robust, he is admonished not to get into fights; when aged and declining in energy, he is admonished not to be greedy.

三棱针 [sān léng zhēn] three-edged needle ~ 法 three-edged needling/ ~ 是一种针刺器具。 Three-edged needle is a kind of acupuncture tool.

三品 [sān pǐn] three grades 药分 ~ :上品、中品和下品。 There are three grades of herbal medicinals: upper, middle and lower.

三阳经 [sān yáng jīng] three yang meridians

三因制宜 [sān yīn zhì yí] three considerations ~ 指因时制宜、因地制宜和因人制宜。 Three considerations refer to environmental consideration, consideration of individual's constitution and consideration of the climatic and seasonal conditions in treatment for diseases.

三阴经 [sān yīn jīng] three yin meridians

散 sǎn

散刺 [sǎn cì] scattered needling ~ 又叫"豹文刺"。 Scattered needling is also known as "leopard-spot needling".

散剂 [sǎn jì] powder medicine

散脉 [sǎn mài] scattered pulse

散 sàn

散步 [sàn bù] walking, taking a walk 久坐宜 ~ 。 It is good to take a walk after long sitting. /最近的研究显示 ~ 激发创造力。 Recent studies suggest that walking bolsters creativity.

散寒 [sàn hán] dissipating cold ~ 除湿 dissipating cold and dampness/ ~ 温肾 dissipating cold and warming the kidney/ ~ 止痛 dissipating cold to kill pain

散结 [sàn jié] disintegrating a mass ~ 通络 disintegrating a mass to dredge meridians/ ~ 消癥 disintegrating an abdominal mass

散饮止呕 [sàn yǐn zhǐ ǒu] removing retained morbid fluid to stop vomiting

散瘀 [sàn yū] dissipating blood stasis ~ 活血 dissipating blood stasis to activate blood circulation ~ 消肿 dissipating blood stasis to subside a swelling

搔 SAO
搔 sāo

搔伤 [sāo shāng] scratch 那只是一点

S

~。That is only a scratch.

搔痒[sāo yǎng] scratching 别再 ~ 了。Stop scratching yourself. /丘疹越 ~ 越厉害。Scratching the rash will make it worse.

色涩啬塞 SE

色 sè

色白入肺[sè bái rù fèi] white acting on the lung

色彩疗法[sè cǎi liáo fǎ] color therapy ~ 的具体应用 application of the color therapy/利用五行生克的原理以确定色彩疗法的治疗原则。The treating principle of the color therapy depends on the theory of sequential generation and restraint among the five phases.

色苍苍[sè cāng cāng] gray complexion ~ 如死状 similar to the complexion of a dead person

色赤入心[sè chì rù xīn] red acting on the heart

色调[sè diào] tone 冷 ~ cold tone/暖 ~ warm tone

色恶不食[sè è bù shí] not eating food with abnormal color

色光浴[sè guāng yù] colored light bath ~ 治疗 treatment with colored light bath

色黑入肾[sè hēi rù shèn] black acting on the kidney

色黄入脾[sè huáng rù pí] yellow acting on the spleen

色青入肝[sè qīng rù gān] dark greyish green acting on the liver

色泽[sè zé] color and luster 望色包括观察面部 ~ 变化。Inspection of the complexion includes observation of the change of the facial color and luster.

色诊[sè zhěn] inspection of the complexion

涩 sè

涩肠[sè cháng] arresting intestinal disorder ~ 药 medicinals that arrest intestinal disorders/ ~ 止泻 arresting diarrhea

涩精[sè jīng] arresting seminal emission 金锁固精丸有 ~ 的功效。*Jinsuo Gujing* Pills work to arrest seminal emission.

涩脉[sè mài] rough pulse 气滞血瘀证常见 ~。Rough pulse is usually found in a pattern of stagnated qi and blood.

啬 sè

啬神[sè shén] feeling calm ~ 以养性 feeling calm to discipline one's temperament

塞 sè

塞兑[sè duì] closing the mouth gently (in *qigong* exercise)

沙砂杀痧 SHA

沙 shā

沙疗法[shā liáo fǎ] sand therapy

沙浴[shā yù] sand bath 自然～natural sand bath

砂 shā
砂皮舌[shā pí shé] sand-paper-like tongue

杀 shā
杀虫[shā chóng] killing worms or parasites ～剂 insecticides/～止痒 killing parasites and relieving itching
杀蛔虫剂[shā huí chóng jì] ascaricide
杀气[shā qì] coolness and coldness in autumn

痧 shā
痧气[shā qì] eruptive disease ～以夏秋季多见。Eruptive disease is usually found in summer and autumn.
痧子[shā zǐ] measles 出～contracting measles

晒 SHAI
晒 shài
晒背[shài bèi] back sunbathing～可补充人体阳气。Back sunbathing supplements yang-qi.

山膻闪疝善 SHAN
山 shān
山根[shān gēn] root of the nose
山岚瘴气[shān lán zhàng qì] mountainous miasma ～常见于岭南一带。Mountainous miasma is often found in the south of the Five Ridges.

膻 shān
膻味[shān wèi] lamb smell 这羊肉太～。The lamb has got a strong smell.

闪 shǎn
闪挫[shǎn cuò] sudden sprain and contusion
闪罐法[shǎn guàn fǎ] flash cupping ～多用于治疗局部肌肉麻木等症。Flash cupping is often applicable to topical muscular numbness.
闪痛[shǎn tòng] sprain pain
闪腰[shǎn yāo] sudden lumbar sprain

疝 shàn
疝[shàn] hernia, lower abdominal colic ～气 hernia

善 shàn
善悲[shàn bēi] easily to be sorrowful 心肝血虚则易。Blood deficiency of the heart and liver easily leads to sorrow.
善饥[shàn jī] easy to feel hungry 常见于消渴。An abnormal increasing hunger is usually found in wasting-thirst disorder. /～而不能食。Although one easily feels hungry, he has no desire for food.
善色[shàn sè] favorable color 若面见～,则病情较轻。A favorable color of the sickly complexion suggests a mild case.
善太息[shàn tài xī] preference for deep sighing 两胁痛,～。When one has hypochondrial pain, he prefers deep signing.
善忘[shàn wàng] amnesia 心脾两虚证可见～。Deficiency in the heart and

spleen leads to amnesia.

善言[shàn yán] good at discussion ~ 古者,必验于今。Those who are good at discussing matters of ancient times must apply them to the present. / ~ 天者,必应于人。Those who are good at explaining the law of Heaven can certainly apply it to human affairs.

善治药者,不如善治食[shàn zhì yào zhě, bù rú shàn zhì shí] It is better to know the knowledge of food than that of medicinals.

伤赏上 SHANG
伤 shāng

伤风[shāng fēng] common cold ~ 咳嗽 coughing in common cold/我 ~ 了。I have had common cold.

伤寒 [shāng hán] cold-induced disease; cold damage; typhoid ~ 表证 exterior pattern of cold-induced disease ~ 亡阳 yang depletion of cold-induced disease/ ~ 蓄水证 cold-induced disease associated wth edema/ ~ 蓄血证 cold-induced disease associated with blood accumulation/ ~ 学派的形成早于温病学派。The School of Cold-induced Disease took shape prior to the School of Warm-pathogen Disease.

伤津[shāng jīn] impairment of body fluids ~ 动血 hemorrhage due to impairment of body fluids/温病血热证后期常有 ~ 动血之症。Hemorrhage due to impairment of body fluids is often found at the late stage of a blood-heat pattern in warm-pathogen disease.

伤筋[shāng jīn] injury to tissue ~ 动骨 injury to tissues and bones

伤酒 [shāng jiǔ] disorder due to drinking too much liquor ~ 恶寒 aversion to cold due to drinking too much liquor/ ~ 头痛 headache due to drinking too much liquor

伤科 [shāng kē] (department of) traumatology ~ 医院 hospital of traumatology/ ~ 是诊治跌打损伤的一门专科。Traumatology is a branch of medicine, particularly dealing with injury from fall and stumble, contusion and strain.

伤口[shāng kǒu] wound ~ 敷料 wound dressing/ ~ 愈合 healing of a wound

伤乳食 [shāng rǔ shí] dyspeptic vomiting and diarrhea

伤乳吐[shāng rǔ tù] infant vomiting

伤食 [shāng shí] impairment due to improper diet 小儿 ~ infantile impairment due to improper food

伤暑 [shāng shǔ] sunstroke; disorder due to summer-heat

伤胃 [shāng wèi] impairment of the stomach 过食寒凉、辛辣均可 ~ 。Impairment of the stomach is caused by much consumption of cold, cool or spicy food.

伤心 [shāng xīn] broken heart;

impairment of the heart 过喜则～。
Overjoy impairs the heart.

伤形 [shāng xíng] impairment of the
body

伤重昏聩 [shāng zhòng hūn kuì] stupor
due to severe injury

赏 shǎng

赏花 [shǎng huā] enjoying flowers ～解
闷 enjoying flowers to relieve
boredom/ ～ 令 人 神 往。 Enjoying
flowers has a strong appeal.

赏 心 悦 目 [shǎng xīn yuè mù]
refreshing for the mind and pleasing to
the eye /西湖的美丽景色 ～。 The
beautiful West Lake scenery is a
refreshing and heartening sight.

赏月 [shǎng yuè] enjoying the moon 全
家中秋 ～。 The family enjoyed a full
bright moon at the Mid-autumn
Festival.

上 shàng

上病下取 [shàng bìng xià qǔ] needling
applied to the lower body to treat
upper disorders

上丹田 [shàng dān tián] upper *Dantian*
习功者多采用意守下丹田,很少意
守上丹田。 The mind is usually
concentrated on the lower *Dantian*,
rather than on the upper *Dantian* in
qigong exercise.

上风头 [shàng fēng tóu] the direction
from which the wind is coming 站在
～ standing on the side where the wind
is coming

上 工 [shàng gōng] good and
experienced physician in ancient
times ～ 不治已病治未病。 Super
physicians put prevention before
disease arising instead of treatment for
occurred disease.

上火 [shàng huǒ] suffering from excessive
internal heat ～牙痛 toothache due to
excessive internal heat

上焦 [shàng jiāo] upper-energizer ～湿
热 dampness-heat in the upper-
energizer/ ～ 如 雾。 The upper-
energizer resembles a sprayer.

上气 [shàng qì] adverse rise of qi ～喘
促 panting due to adverse rise of qi

上窍 [shàng qiào] orifice on the face

上实下虚 [shàng shí xià xū] upper
excess and lower deficiency

上吐下泻 [shàng tù xià xiè] vomiting
and diarrhea ～ 多 见 于 霍 乱 病。
Severe vomiting and diarrhea are often
found in choleraic turmoil.

上脘 [shàng wǎn] epigastrium 食积气
逆, ～ 胀 闷 不 适。 Indigestion and
adverse rise of qi lead to fullness and
discomfort in the epigastrium.

上下配穴 [shàng xià pèi xué] combination
of the upper and lower acupoints

上虚下实 [shàng xū xià shí] upper
deficiency and lower excess

烧少 SHAO
烧 shāo

烧存性 [shāo cún xìng] nature-preservative burning

烧山火［shāo shān huǒ］mountain-burning-fire method ~ 在临床上很少用，只用于急救。The mountain-burning-fire method is rarely used except in emergency treatment.

烧针法［shāo zhēn fǎ］needling with a heated needle ~ 是治疗寒邪为病的有效方法。Needling with a heated needle is an effective method for diseases due to cold.

少 shǎo

少气［shǎo qì］insufficiency of qi ~ 不足以息 shortness of breath due to lack of qi/ ~ 懒言 disinclination to talk due to lack of qi/ ~ 可因脏气虚弱，尤以肺气虚损，中气不足为常见。Lack of qi presents in insufficient qi of the zang-organs, especially the lung and middle-energizer.

少神［shǎo shén］lack of vitality

少食多餐［shǎo shí duō cān］having more meals a day but a little food at each time 糖尿病人宜 ~。Diabetics should have more meals a day but a little food at each time.

少私寡欲［shǎo sī guǎ yù］having no selfishness and desires ~ 者 a person with few worldly desires/ ~ , 知足常乐。Without selfishness and desires contentment brings happiness.

少思以养神［shǎo sī yǐ yǎng shén］mental relaxation achieved by less pondering

少 shào

少白头［shào bái tóu］young person with greying hair

少不勤行［shào bù qín xíng］not excessively fond of having good time in childhood ~ , 壮不竞时，长而安贫，……养生之方也。A person is neither excessively fond of having a good time in childhood nor seeking instant success and quick profits when young, and he is happy to live a simple life in middle age... This is the sound strategy for health preservation.

少阳人［shào yáng rén］*Shaoyang*-featured person

少阴人［shào yīn rén］*Shaoyin*-featured person

舌蛇舍社摄麝 SHE

舌 shé

舌本［shé běn］body of the tongue

舌边［shé biān］margin of the tongue ~ 红 red margin of the tongue ~ 有齿痕，主脾虚湿盛。The tooth-printed margin on the tongue indicates deficiency in the spleen and excessive dampness.

舌淡［shé dàn］pale tongue ~ 无苔主气阴不足。Pale tongue without coating indicates deficiency of qi and yin.

舌抵上颚［shé dǐ shàng è］sticking the tongue against the palate

舌根［shé gēn］root of the tongue

舌尖[shé jiān] tip of the tongue

舌謇[shé jiǎn] sluggish tongue

舌绛[shé jiàng]deep-red tongue

舌强[shé jiàng]rigid tongue

舌色[shé sè] tongue color 望~是舌诊的重要内容之一。Inspection of the tongue color is an important way in evaluation of the tongue.

舌苔[shé tāi] tongue coating; fur ~ 黏腻 slimy and greasy fur/ ~ 薄白主外寒。Thin white fur implies an exterior cold pattern.

舌象[shé xiàng] tongue manifestation 临床上~比较复杂,不能简单地归类。Clinically, tongue manifestations are complicated, so they are not simply classified.

舌心[shé xīn] center of the tongue

舌形[shé xíng] shape of the tongue

舌针疗法[shé zhēn liáo fǎ] tongue acupuncture therapy

舌诊[shé zhěn] tongue diagnosis ~ 包括观舌质,查舌苔和看舌态。Tongue diagnosis involves inspection of the texture, coating and shape of the tongue.

蛇 shé

蛇丹[shé dān]herps zoster

蛇毒[shé dú] snake venom ~ 内攻 inward attack by snake venom

蛇头疔[shé tóu dīng]felon

舍 shě

舍脉从症[shě mài cóng zhèng] observing symptoms rather than the pulse quality

舍症从脉[shě zhèng cóng mài] observing the pulse quality rather than symptoms

社 shè

社会医学[shè huì yī xué] social medicine

摄 shè

摄生[shè shēng] keeping healthy, keeping fit ~ 学 eubiotics/ ~ 之道 way to keep fit

摄影[shè yǐng] photography ~ 师 photographer/职业 ~ professional photography/真正优秀的 ~ 作品是能够传达情感的。A genuine photo conveys affection.

麝 shè

麝香[shè xiāng] musk ~ 辛温,入心、脾、肝经。Musk, warm in nature, acts on the Heart, Spleen and Liver meridians.

伸身深神审肾慎 SHEN

伸 shēn

伸舌[shēn shé] sticking out one's tongue ~ 时,必须自然地把舌伸出口外。The tongue should stick out naturally.

伸腰沉胯[shēn yāo chén kuà] stretching the lower back and keeping the hips sunk

伸足卧[shēn zú wò] sleeping with legs stretched ~ 一身俱暖。Sleeping with legs stretched makes the body warm.

身 shēn

身不仁［shēn bù rén］general numbness

身寒［shēn hán］feeling cold 阳气不足不能温煦机体则 ~ 。Failure of the body to be warmed due to deficient yang-qi results in a feeling of cold.

身热［shēn rè］fever ~ 不解 unrelieved fever/ ~ 不扬 low grade fever/ ~ 烦心 fever with vexation/ ~ 汗出 fever with sweating

身心［shēn xīn］body and mind ~ 健康 psychosomatic health

身心医学［shēn xīn yī xué］psychosomatic medicine

身痒［shēn yǎng］itching

身重［shēn zhòng］heaviness sensation of the body and limbs 湿热困阻,阳气不能畅达, 则身重。Fettered by dampness-heat, yang-qi fails to circulate smoothly, resulting in a feeling of heaviness in the body and limbs.

深 shēn

深呼吸［shēn hū xī］deep breathing ~ 有益健康。Deep breathing is good for health.

神 shén

神［shén］vitality; mental activity; spirit ~ 不安啼 infantile restlessness/ ~ 不守舍 out of one's mind, spirit failing to keep to its abode/ ~ 志不清 in a confused state of mind/得 ~ 者昌,失 ~ 者亡。Presence of vitality indicates favorable prognosis, while loss of vitality leads to poor prognosis.

神呆少言［shén dāi shǎo yán］blank expression and taciturnity ~ 为失神之证。A blank expression and taciturnity indicate loss of vitality.

神光［shén guāng］expression in (one's) eyes ~ 充沛 bright eyes/ ~ 耗散 lusterless and spiritless eyes/ ~ 自现 photopsia/神既失守, ~ 不聚。If one's spirit fails to keep to its abode, he will lose the expression in the eyes.

神静［shén jìng］quietude ~ 则气血流通。Quietude leads to smooth flow of qi and blood.

神劳［shén láo］mental exhaustion ~ 多因情志过极、思虑过度等所致。Mental exhaustion is mostly caused by emotional stress and worry beyond measure.

神乱［shén luàn］mental disorder; mental disturbance ~ 临床表现为焦虑恐惧、狂躁不安、淡漠痴呆等。The clinical manifestations of mental disorders are anxiety and fear, manic agitation, indifferent expression and dementia, etc.

神满者［shén mǎn zhě］vigorous person

神明［shén míng］mental activity ~ 失守 disturbed mental activity/心主 ~ The heart governs the mental activity.

神气充足［shén qì chōng zú］full of vitality 只有 ~ ,人体的功能才能旺盛而协调。Only when one is full of vitality can the body function actively and work efficiently.

神强必多寿［shén qiáng bì duō shòu］One with full vitality enjoys a long life.

神清气和［shén qīng qì hé］mentally clear and emotionally peaceful

神情［shén qíng］expression

神散［shén sàn］dispersed spirit ~ 则气消。Dispersed spirit results in qi consumption.

神志［shén zhì］consciousness ~ 不清 in a confused state of mind/ ~ 清醒 in a clear state of mind

审 shěn

审因施治［shěn yīn shī zhì］cause determination and treatment

审证求因［shěn zhèng qiú yīn］cause-seeking from symptoms

肾 shèn

肾病禁甘［shèn bìng jìn gān］sweet abstained in patients with kidney problems

肾［shèn］kidney ~ 藏精 essence stored in the kidney/ ~ 藏志 kidney storing will

肾不纳气［shèn bù nà qì］failure of the kidney to grasp qi

肾间动气［shèn jiān dòng qì］motive qi between kidneys

肾精［shèn jīng］kidney-essence ~ 不足 insufficient kidney-essence/ ~ 不足则男子精少不育，女子经闭不孕。Insufficient kidney-essence may lead to sterility due to oligospermia and amenorrhea.

肾经［shèn jīng］Kidney Meridian

肾开窍于二阴［shèn kāi qiào yú èr yīn］urethra and anus being the specific openings of the kidney

肾开窍于耳［shèn kāi qiào yú ěr］ear, the window of the kidney

肾气［shèn qì］kidney-qi ~ 不固 insecurity of kidney-qi/ ~ 盛 abundant kidney-qi/ ~ 虚 deficiency of kidney-qi/女子七岁，~ 盛 abundant kidney-qi in girls at the age of seven

肾为水之下源［shèn wéi shuǐ zhī xià yuán］kidney, the lower source of water

肾为先天之本［shèn wéi xiān tiān zhī běn］kidney, the root of the human innate ability

肾虚［shèn xū］deficiency in the kidney ~ 耳鸣 tinnitus due to deficiency in the kidney/ ~ 水泛 edema due to deficiency in the kidney/ ~ 眩晕 dizziness due to deficiency in the kidney/ ~ 阳痿 impotence due to deficiency in the kidney/治疗 ~ 崩漏宜补肾益精，强冲脉。To treat metrorrhagia and metrostaxis due to deficiency in the kidney, it is necessary to vitalize the kidney and replenish its essence, and strengthen the Thoroughfare Vessel.

肾主骨［shèn zhǔ gǔ］bones dominated by the kidney

S

肾主纳气 [shèn zhǔ nà qì] kidney governing qi grasping

肾主生殖 [shèn zhǔ shēng zhí] kidney governing reproduction

肾主水液 [shèn zhǔ shuǐ yè] kidney governing water

肾主先天 [shèn zhǔ xiān tiān] kidney governing the innate ability

肾子 [shèn zǐ] testis

慎 shèn

慎独 [shèn dú] self-discipline when alone ~ 思想 the thought of self-discipline when alone/ ~ 是儒家传统的美德之一。 Self-discipline when alone is one of the traditional virtues of Confucianism.

慎起居 [shèn qǐ jū] leading a regular life ~ , 节饮食, 适寒暑 leading a regular life, having proper diet and adapting oneself to summer and winter/ ~ 养生法 health preservation by leading a regular life

慎味 [shèn wèi] avoiding surfeit of food and drink 节劳 ~ 养精。 Never work too hard, avoid surfeit of food and drink, and preserve essence.

升生声省圣胜盛 SHENG

升 shēng

升补 [shēng bǔ] tonifying with medicinals that ascend yang-qi 立春 ~ 。 Once spring sets in, it is essential to build up health with medicinals that ascend yang-qi.

升发 [shēng fā] elevating

升降出入 [shēng jiàng chū rù] ascending, descending, exiting and entering ~ , 无器不有。 All the organs have the ascending, descending, exiting and entering functions.

升降浮沉 [shēng jiàng fú chén] ascending, descending, floating and sinking 草药都有 ~ 四气。 All medicinal herbs have four properties—ascending, descending, floating and sinking.

升降息则气立孤危 [shēng jiàng xī zé qì lì gū wēi] Stop of ascending and descending of yin and yang causes qi collapse.

升清降浊 [shēng qīng jiàng zhuó] ascending the usables and descending the unusables ~ 是人体正常生理功能的体现和概括。 Ascending the usables and descending the unusables are the normal physiological functions of the body.

升阳 [shēng yáng] ascending yang ~ 举陷 ascending yang to cure sagging/ ~ 透疹 ascending yang to induce eruptions

生 shēng

生化 [shēng huà] production and transformation ~ 收藏 production, transformation, collection and storage

生克制化 [shēng kè zhì huà] sequential generation and restraint among the five phases

生猛海鲜[shēng měng hǎi xiān] fresh seafood

生气[shēng qì] active qi; invigorating vitality ~之源 source of qi

生气通天[shēng qì tōng tiān] yang-qi going up to Heaven

生生化化[shēng shēng huà huà] incessant changes and variations in nature

生药[shēng yào] crude drug ~家 pharmacognosist/ ~学 pharmacognosy

生长壮老已[shēng zhǎng zhuàng lǎo yǐ] newborn, growing, robust, aged and deceased

生殖[shēng zhí] reproduction ~之精 essence for reproduction

声 shēng

声带[shēng dài] vocal cord ~发炎，不适当的发声或说话过多易使~疲劳。Fatigue of the vocal cord is caused by its inflammation, improper phonation or talking too much.

声嘶[shēng sī] hoarseness ~力竭 hoarse and exhausted

声重[shēng zhòng] deep and harsh voice 肺肾不交则~。Breakdown of the normal physiological coordination between the lung and kidney leads to deep and harsh voice.

省 shěng

省心[shěng xīn] no worry

省言[shěng yán] talking less ~以养气。Talk less in order to nurture qi.

圣 shèng

圣人[shèng rén] sage; excellent physician ~陈阴阳，筋脉和同。Sages who know how to keep fit focus on the regulation of yin and yang, so that the sinews, vessels and bones are strong. / ~春夏养阳，秋冬阳阴，以从其根。Excellent physicians who understand how to keep fit follow the basic principle by replenishing yang-qi in spring and summer and yin-qi in autumn and winter to preserve healthy qi. / ~为无为之事。Sages do things that follow the laws of nature. / ~行之，愚者佩之。The knowledgeable people follow it and the ignorant people oppose it.

胜 shèng

胜形则寿[shèng xíng zé shòu] enjoying a long life when there are abundant essence, qi and vigor even though not strong in physique ~，形胜气则夭。One would enjoy a long life when there are abundant essence and vigor, even though not strong in physique, or one would die young if he cares more about his health than his essence, qi and vigor.

盛 shèng

盛人[shèng rén] obese person

盛衰[shèng shuāi] excess and deficiency

盛则泻之[shèng zé xiè zhī] reducing in

S

an excess condition

尸失诗湿十时石实食使世视拭室舐嗜 SHI

尸 shī

尸厥[shī jué] loss of consciousness

失 shī

失精家 [shī jīng jiā] patient with frequent seminal emission

失眠[shī mián] insomnia, sleeplessness

失饪不食[shī rèn bù shí] never eating poor cooked food

失神[shī shén] loss of vitality ~ 者亡 Loss of vitality is a sign of a critical condition.

失音[shī yīn] aphonia

诗 shī

诗词歌赋[shī cí gē fù] poetry, rhymed verse, song and prose-poetry

诗书悦心 [shī shū yuè xīn] heart pleased by poetry

湿 shī

湿[shī] dampness ~ 痹 arthralgia due to dampness/ ~ 气 dampness/ ~ 邪 pathogenic dampness

湿疮[shī chuāng] eczema

湿毒[shī dú] toxic dampness ~ 内攻 inward attack by toxic dampness/清解 ~ removing toxic dampness

湿火[shī huǒ] dampness-fire

湿剂 [shī jì] formula that removes dampness 清热利 ~ formulas that clear heat and dampness

湿家[shī jiā] patient usually presenting a dampness pattern

湿冷[shī lěng] damp and chilly

湿热 [shī rè] dampness-heat ~ 互结 union of dampness and heat/ ~ 内蕴 internal retention of dampness-heat

湿热质 [shī rè zhì] type of dampness-heat constitution ~ 需清化湿热。It is advisable to clear dampness and heat for people with the dampness-heat constitution.

湿伤脾阳[shī shāng pí yáng] dampness impairing kidney-yang

湿胜则濡下 [shī shèng zé rú xià] excessive dampness causing diarrhea

湿痰[shī tán] dampness-phlegm ~ 流注 metastatic abscess due to dampness-heat/ ~ 阻络 meridians obstructed by dampness-phlegm

湿温 [shī wēn] dampness and warm-pathogen ~ 病 disease caused by dampness and warm-pathogen

湿疹 [shī zhěn] eczema 面颈部 ~ faciocervical eczema

十 shí

十八反 [shí bā fǎn] eighteen incompatibilities《本草》明言 ~ 。 *Shen Nong's Herbal Classic* states the eighteen incompatibilities of Chinese herbal medicinals.

十二经脉 [shí èr jīng mài] twelve meridians

十九畏 [shí jiǔ wèi] nineteen antagonisms 中药十八反, ~ 。There

are eighteen incompatibilities and nineteen antagonisms of Chinese herbal medicinals.

十问[shí wèn] ten questions ~ 歌 verse of the ten questions

十五络脉［shí wǔ luò mài］fifteen collaterals

时 shí

时病[shí bìng] seasonal disease

时不可违[shí bù kě wéi] seizing the time

时辰[shí chén] one of the 12 two-hour periods ~ 用药 taking herbal medicinals according to different periods of time during a day

时方[shí fāng] formulas developed after Zhang Zhongjing's period

时寒时热［shí hán shí rè］alternative chills and fever

时间治疗学［shí jiān zhì liáo xué］chronotherapeutics

时令[shí lìng] season ~ 变化 seasonal changes/ ~ 病 seasonal disease/ ~ 不正 unseasonal weather/正当 ~ being in season

时邪［shí xié］ seasonal pathogenic factors

时疫［shí yì］ epidemic ~ 痢 toxic dysentery

石 shí

石瘕[shí jiǎ] hard uterine mass

石疽[shí jū] stony nodule

石淋[shí lìn] stone stranguria

石女[shí nǚ] women with hypoplastic vagina

实 shí

实喘［shí chuǎn］panting in an excess condition

实脉[shí mài] full pulse ~ 主实证。 Full pulse suggests an excess pattern.

实则泻其子［shí zé xiè qí zǐ］treating an excess pattern by reducing pathogenic factors of its child-organ

实证[shí zhèng] excess pattern

实中夹虚［shí zhōng jiā xū］excess pattern accompanied by a deficiency pattern

食 shí

食饱不可睡［shí bǎo bù kě shuì］never going to bed immediately after having a heavy meal ~ ,睡则诸疾生。Never go to bed immediately after having a heavy meal, otherwise, diseases will follow.

食补[shí bǔ] eating nutritious food 药补不如 ~ 。One 'd rather eat nutritious food than taking tonics. /正常的身体功能下降以 ~ 为主。 Emphasis should be placed on eating more nutritious food when there occurs lowered functioning of the body.

食不甘味［shí bù gān wèi］having no appetite 寝不安席, ~ sleeplessness and loss of appetite due to worry beyond measure

食不化[shí bù huà] indigestion

食不下［shí bù xià］difficult to take food ~ 者,胃脘隔也。Difficulty of

S

taking food is due to obstruction of the stomach.

食不语[shí bù yǔ] not talking at meals

食不欲杂[shí bù yù zá] not eating miscellaneous food at a meal

食复[shí fù] relapse due to improper diet

食后养生[shí hòu yǎng shēng] care taken after meals ~ 包括漱口、散步和按摩等活动。Care taken after meals includes rinsing the mouth, taking a walk and doing massage.

食借药力[shí jiè yào lì] action of herbal medicinals strengthened with the help of food ~，药助食威 action of herbal medicinals strengthened with the help of food and mutual assistance between food and medicinals

食厥[shí jué] crapulent syncope due to indigestion 小儿风热食积壅滞可酿成 ~。Children attacked by wind and heat may develop crapulent syncope due to indigestion.

食疗 [shí liáo] dietary therapy, dietotherapy ~ 方 formula for dietary therapy/ ~ 不愈，然后命药。When dietotherapy fails, medicinal treatment follows.

食气[shí qì] taking in qi

食肉则复[shí ròu zé fù] relapse from eating meat

食膳以疗[shí shàn yǐ liáo] treatment helped by dietotherapy

食少便溏[shí shǎo biàn táng] poor appetite and loose feces 脾胃虚弱之人，~。People suffering from lowered functioning of the spleen and stomach have poor appetite and excrete loose feces.

食调[shí tiáo] improving health by diet regulation

食无求饱[shí wú qiú bǎo] not eating a big meal 君子 ~，居无求安。A gentleman does not seek a big meal and leads a life of ease and comfort.

食物 [shí wù] food ~ 中毒 food poisoning

食医[shí yī] dietitian in ancient times

食饮[shí yǐn] nutritious food and drink ~ 者,热无灼灼,寒无沧沧。寒温中适，故气将持，乃不致邪僻也。In terms of diet, it should be warm but not overly hot; it should be cold but not overly cold. Healthy qi can be conserved internally only when the temperature is moderate. This also prevents the invasion by pathogenic factors and disease.

食欲[shí yù] appetite ~ 不振 having poor appetite/ ~ 过盛 having a robust appetite

食远服[shí yuǎn fú] taking medicines between meals

食治 [shí zhì] dietary therapy, dietotherapy 用 ~ 方法防治糖尿病。Dietotherapy is an alternative in prevention and treatment for diabetes.

食滞[shí zhì] indigestion ~ 脘痛

stomachache due to indigestion

食滞胃脘［shí zhì wèi wǎn］food retained in the stomach

食中［shí zhòng］stroke due to surfeit

使 shǐ

使药［shǐ yào］guide medicinal

世 shì

世医［shì yī］lineage of physicians

视 shì

视觉疲劳［shì jué pí láo］visual fatigue 自我按摩可缓解 ~。Self-massage can relieve visual fatigue.

视物模糊［shì wù mó hū］blurred vision ~常见于久病或年老体弱之人。Blurred vision is often found in patients with chronic disease, the aged or people of poor health. / ~ 多由肝肾亏虚，精血不足，目失充养而致。Blurred vision is due to lowered functioning of the liver and kidney and deficiency of essence and blood, which fails to nourish the eyes.

拭 shì

拭目［shì mù］covering eyes with warm hands ~以待。Wait and see.

室 shì

室温［shì wēn］indoor temperature ~调节 regulation of indoor temperature

室女［shì nǚ］virgin

舐 shì

舐颚［shì è］licking the upper jaw

嗜 shì

嗜偏食［shì piān shí］predilection for some food

嗜食异物［shì shí yì wù］preference for eating things other than food 小儿虫积，多 ~。Children with malnutrition due to parasite infestation may have preference for eating things other than food.

嗜睡［shì shuì］somnolence 湿邪侵犯人体，头中如裹, ~ 人昏蒙。When the body is invaded by pathogenic dampness, there may occur such symptoms as feeling of tightly bandaged head, drowsiness and dizzy spells.

嗜欲［shì yù］desire for the satisfaction of the sense/ ~ 不同 differed partiality and interest/ ~ 不能劳其目。Improper addiction and avarice could not distract their eyes.

嗜欲不止［shì yù bù zhǐ］desires out of control 私心太重, ~ too much selfishness and desires out of control

收手守寿瘦 SHOU

收 shōu

收藏［shōu cáng］collection ~ 家collector/ ~ 品 collection/ ~ 文物 collecting antiques/博物馆里 ~ 大批文物。The museum has a large collection of antiques.

收功［shōu gōng］ending exercise in *qigong*

收敛神气［shōu liǎn shén qì］gathering the scattering mind ~, 使秋气平。

Gather the scattering mind to allow the body to adapt to the autumn air and achieve balance.

收敛生肌[shōu liǎn shēng jī] making astringency and promoting tissue regeneration

收涩[shōu sè] arresting discharge ~ 药 astringents/ ~ 止血 hemostasis with medicinals/ ~ 止遗 checking seminal emission

收臀松膝[shōu tún sōng xī] contracting the buttocks and relaxing the knees

手 shǒu

手法[shǒu fǎ] manipulation, maneuver ~ 操作 manipulations/ ~ 复位术 manual reduction/ ~ 牵引 manual traction

手炉[shǒu lú] hand warmer

手气[shǒu qì] luck

手巧[shǒu qiǎo] deft 心灵 ~ clever and deft

手腕[shǒu wàn] wrist ~ 疼痛 wrist pain/转动 ~ turning wrist

手小腹相叠[shǒu xiǎo fù xiāng dié] letting hands overlap one another on the lower abdomen

手艺[shǒu yì] craftsmanship

手印[shǒu yìn] hand gesture

手针[shǒu zhēn] hand acupuncture ~ 疗法 hand acupuncture therapy/ ~ 麻醉 hand acupuncture analgesia

手指[shǒu zhǐ] finger ~ 麻木 numbness of fingers/ ~ 伤筋 injury to a finger

手足皲裂[shǒu zú cūn liè] chapped hands and feet 燥邪伤阴,肌肤失养, ~ 。 Chapped hands and feet are caused by failure of the skin and muscles to be nourished when yin is impaired by dryness.

手足心热[shǒu zú xīn rè] feverish feeling in the palms and soles

守 shǒu

守旧[shǒu jiù] sticking to old ways ~ 派 fogey

守一[shǒu yī] single-mindedness 道家养生主张 ~ 、坐忘、内视。For health preservation Taoists developed ways such as single-mindedness, sitting oblivion and inward vision to cultivate oneself.

寿 shòu

寿[shòu] lifespan 上 ~ long lifespan (100 years of age or more)/中 ~ intermediate lifespan (80 to 100 years of age)/下 ~ short lifespan (under the age of 80)/茶 ~ "tea" lifespan (108 years of age)

寿斑[shòu bān] age spot

寿敝天地[shòu bì tiān dì] life expectancy as long as that of Heaven and Earth

寿辰[shòu chén] birthday

寿面[shòu miàn] longevity noodles

寿命[shòu mìng] lifespan 预期 ~ average expectancy

瘦 shòu

瘦薄舌[shòu báo shé] thin tongue

瘦人[shòu rén] thin person ~ 火多

Skinny people usually have much fire.

书舒疏熟暑蜀数腧术漱 SHU

书 shū

书法［shū fǎ］calligraphy ~ 家 calligrapher/ ~ 养生 health preservation with calligraphy/中国 ~ 不仅注重写字的技巧也注重培养人的品格。Chinese calligraphy focuses not only on methods of writing but also on cultivating one's character.

舒 shū

舒筋活络［shū jīn huó luò］relaxing muscles and tendons and activating meridians ~，理气止痛 relaxing muscles and tendons and activating meridians to promote smooth flow of qi to kill pain

舒筋通络［shū jīn tōng luò］relaxing muscles and tendons and dredging meridians ~ 有利于损伤组织的修复。Relaxing muscles and tendons and dredging meridians are beneficial to helping repairment of the injured tissues. / ~ 治疗的着眼点就是针对疼痛和肌紧张这两方面。The therapy of relaxing muscles and tendons and dredging meridians focuses on two aspects：relieving pain and muscular contraction.

舒心［shū xīn］contended

舒腰松腹［shū yāo sōng fù］keeping the lower back and abdomen relaxed

舒展［shū zhǎn］extending ~ 筋骨 stretching one's muscles and joints

疏 shū

疏涤［shū dí］cleansing ~ 五脏。Stagnation in the five *zang*-organs is cleansed.

疏风［shū fēng］dissipating wind ~ 散寒解表 dissipating wind-cold to release an exterior pattern/ ~ 透疹 dissipating wind and promoting eruptions（as in measles）/ ~ 泄热 dissipating wind and clearing heat/ ~ 止痉 dissipating wind to arrest convulsion

疏肝［shū gān］soothing the liver ~ 解郁 soothing the liver to remove stagnancy of liver-qi/ ~ 理气，缓急止痛 soothing the liver to regulate its qi flow and relieve spasm and pain

疏散风寒［shū sàn fēng hán］dissipating wind-cold 外感风寒表证，治宜 ~。It is necessary to dissipate wind-cold in an exterior pattern due to wind-cold.

疏散风热［shū sàn fēng rè］dissipating wind-heat ~ 治疗外感风热之证。Dissipating wind-heat is an approach used in treatment for an exterior pattern due to wind-heat.

疏松［shū sōng］relieved and relaxed

疏通［shū tōng］dredging ~ 经脉 dredging meridians/ ~ 气血 promoting smooth flow of qi and blood

疏泄［shū xiè］dispersing 肝主 ~ smooth flow of qi ruled by the liver

S

熟 shú

熟菜［shú cài］cooked dish

熟食［shú shí］cooked food

熟水［shú shuǐ］boiled water

熟油［shú yóu］boiled oil

暑 shǔ

暑风［shǔ fēng］summer-heat wind

暑伏［shǔ fú］beginning of the hottest days of the year

暑热［shǔ rè］summer-heat ~ 动风 stirring of internal wind due to summer-heat/ ~ 症 disease due to summer-heat

暑痧［shǔ shā］heat stroke with vomiting and diarrhea

暑湿［shǔ shī］summer-heat and dampness ~ 感冒 common cold due to summer-heat and dampness

暑温［shǔ wēn］summer warm-pathogen 外感 ~ 之邪 exposure to summer warm-pathogens

蜀 shǔ

蜀犬吠日［shǔ quǎn fèi rì］making fuss about small things

数 shǔ

数九［shǔ jiǔ］beginning of the coldest days of the year ~ 寒天 the coldest days of the year

数息［shǔ xī］breath counting

腧 shù

腧穴［shù xué］acupoint ~ 特异性 specific characteristics of acupoints

术 shù

术数［shù shù］ways to cultivate health 法于阴阳, 和于 ~。Follow the rule of yin and yang and adjust the methods of keeping fit.

漱 shù

漱津［shù jīn］gargling with saliva ~ 咽唾 gargling the mouth with saliva and swallowing it

漱口［shù kǒu］rinsing the mouth; gargling ~ 剂 gargle/用盐水 ~。Gargle with salt water./食毕常 ~ 预防龋齿。Gargling after meals prevents decayed teeth.

刷耍 SHUA

刷 shuā

刷牙［shuā yá］brushing teeth 睡前 ~ brushing teeth before bedtime

耍 shuǎ

耍心眼儿［shuǎ xīn yǎn er］showing off petty tricks

衰 SHUAI

衰 shuāi

衰老［shuāi lǎo］old and feeble 他父亲年过八十, 但不 ~。His father is over 80, but he shows no old and feeble signs.

衰朽［shuāi xiǔ］aged and weakened ~ 残年 declining years

衰之以属［shuāi zhī yǐ shǔ］treating a disease according to its nature

涮 SHUAN

涮 shuàn

涮锅[shuàn guō] hotpot

涮羊肉[shuàn yáng ròu] instant-boiled lamb slices（in a hotpot）, having lamb hotpot

霜双 SHUANG

霜 shuāng

霜降[shuāng jiàng] Frost's Descent

双 shuāng

双脚分开[shuāng jiǎo fēn kāi] standing with feet parallel and flat on the floor

双身[shuāng shēn] pregnancy

双手进针法[shuāng shǒu jìn zhēn fǎ] needle insertion with both hands

双手攀足势[shuāng shǒu pān zú shì] grasping one's feet with hands

双手托天势[shuāng shǒu tuō tiān shì] hands pushing upward

双手握拳[shuāng shǒu wò quán] locking fingers in bear grip

水睡 SHUI

水 shuǐ

水道[shuǐ dào] water passage ~不通 obstruction of the water passage/ ~不利 impaired water passage/肾阳虚, 膀胱气化不利, ~不通, 排尿困难。Deficiency of kidney-yang causes disorder of the qi activity of the urinary bladder, leading to impaired water passage and dysuria.

水痘[shuǐ dòu] chicken pox

水毒[shuǐ dú] disease caused by polluted water

水飞法[shuǐ fēi fǎ] aqueous trituration ~制药法 medicament prepared by aqueous trituration

水谷[shuǐ gǔ] drinks and foods ~精微 essence of drinks and foods/ ~之道 throat/ ~之海 reservoir of drinks and foods, stomach/ ~之气 essence of drinks and foods/人以 ~ 为本。Life depends on drinks and foods.

水罐法[shuǐ guàn fǎ] hydro-cupping

水果冻[shuǐ guǒ dòng] fruit jelly

水火不济[shuǐ huǒ bù jì] disharmony between water phase（kidney）and fire phase（heart）

水煎服[shuǐ jiān fú] taking herbal decoction ~, 一日两次。Take the herbal decoction, twice a day.

水晶包[shuǐ jīng bāo] steamed bread stuffed with sweet lard

水酒[shuǐ jiǔ] watery wine

水逆[shuǐ nì] vomiting of water

水气凌心[shuǐ qì líng xīn] attack of the heart by retained water

水上运动[shuǐ shàng yùn dòng] aquatic sports ~ 能强身健体。Aquatic sports are good for health.

水土[shuǐ tǔ] natural environment

水土不服[shuǐ tǔ bù fú] failure to acclimatize to a new environment ~时 会有呕吐、腹泻等情况出现。When one fails to acclimatize to a new

S

environment, he may throw up, have diarrhea and so on.

水丸[shuǐ wán] watered pill

水乡[shuǐ xiāng] region of rivers and lakes

水泻[shuǐ xiè] watery diarrhea

水形人[shuǐ xíng rén] water-featured person ~主要病在火行,包括心、小肠、血脉等。Water-featured people often suffer from disorders of the fire phase(heart) manifested itself as the problems of the heart, small intestine and vessels.

水郁折之[shuǐ yù zhé zhī] retained fluid removed by drainage

水源洁净[shuǐ yuán jié jìng] clean drinking water ~是居处选择的重要标准。Having clean drinking water is a significant element for choosing a dwelling place.

水曰润下[shuǐ yuē rùn xià] water tending to flow downward

水针[shuǐ zhēn] acupoint injection ~疗法 acupoint injection therapy

水质[shuǐ zhì] water quality 这地区~不好。This area has poor water quality.

水肿[shuǐ zhǒng] edema

睡 shuì

睡不饱饥[shuì bù bǎo jī] not sleeping on an empty or a full stomach

睡功[shuì gōng] *qigong* for sound sleep

睡懒觉[shuì lǎn jiào] getting up late

睡意[shuì yì] sleepiness

睡姿[shuì zī] sleeping pose 古今医家多选择右侧卧为最佳~。Ancient and modern doctors mostly believe sleeping on the right side is the best pose.

睡作狮子卧[shuì zuò shī zi wò] sleeping in lion's pose

顺 SHUN
顺 shùn

顺传[shùn chuán] normal transmission

顺口[shùn kǒu] agreeable to one's taste 这汤真~。The soup is really tasty.

顺气[shùn qì] bringing down adverse flow of lung-qi or stomach-qi ~开郁 bringing down adverse flow of qi and relieving qi stagnation

顺四时而适寒暑[shùn sì shí ér shì hán shǔ] adapting oneself to the weather change in four seasons

顺天因时[shùn tiān yīn shí] following the natural law

顺心[shùn xīn] satisfactory 不~ unsatisfactory

顺应时令[shùn yìng shí lìng] adaptation to seasonal changes

顺应四时[shùn yìng sì shí] adaptation to changes of four seasons

顺应自然[shùn yìng zì rán] following the tide of nature

顺证[shùn zhèng] favorable case ~预后佳。A favorable case often has good prognosis. /脉证相符,多为

~。In a favorable case the pulse quality and pattern are generally matched.

朔数 SHUO

朔 shuò

朔日［shuò rì］first day of each month of the traditional Chinese calendar

朔望［shuò wàng］the first and fifteenth day of each month of the traditional Chinese calendar

朔月［shuò yuè］new moon

数 shuò

数脉［shuò mài］rapid pulse 沉 ~ 主里热。Oeep and rapid pulse suggests internal heat.

司思四 SI

司 sī

司外揣内［sī wài chuǎi nèi］judging the inside by observation of the outside

司药［sī yào］pharmacist

思 sī

思 ［sī］pensiveness ~ 伤脾 Pensiveness impairs the spleen. / ~ 则气结。Pensiveness generates qi stuckness.

思不出位 ［sī bù chū wèi］not considering things outside one's position 曾子曰："君子 ~ "。Zeng Zi, an ancient philosopher said, "A gentleman, in his thoughts, does not go out of his place."

思虑过度［sī lù guò dù］worry beyond measure ~，耗伤心脾。Hard thinking may injure and exhaust the heart and spleen.

思色法［sī sè fǎ］color imagination ~ 有制恐和有利思维的功效。Color imagination is good for controlling terror and improving the faculty of thinking.

思则气结［sī zé qì jié］qi stuckness caused by pensiveness

四 sì

四海［sì hǎi］four reservoirs（seas）

四季养生［sì jì yǎng shēng］health preservation in four seasons

四脚八叉［sì jiǎo bā chā］lying on one's back with arms and legs stretched out 他 ~ 地躺着。He lay on his back with arms and legs stretched out.

四气［sì qì］four properties of herbal medicinals ~ 五味 four properties and five flavors of herbal medicinals

四时［sì shí］four seasons ~ 不正之气 abnormal climate in four seasons/ ~ 行焉，百物兴焉。When four seasons run as usual, everything grows naturally.

四时八节［sì shí bā jié］four seasons and eight solar terms

四体书［sì tǐ shū］four scripts：regular script, cursive script, official script and seal script

S

四维相代[sì wéi xiāng dài] alternative attack of the human body by seasonal pathogenic factors

四言诗[sì yán shī] four-character verse

四诊[sì zhěn] four examinations ~ 合参 analysis of the data obtained from the four examinations

四肢赢弱[sì zhī léi ruò] weak limbs 面色萎黄，~ sallow complexion and weak limbs

松送 SONG

松 sōng

松筋解凝[sōng jīn jiě níng] relaxing muscles and tendons to relieve joint adhesion

松颈[sōng jǐng] relaxing the neck ~ 沉肩 relaxing the neck and shoulders

松静功[sōng jìng gōng] relaxation *qigong* ~ 有调理气机, 疏通经络的功效。The relaxation *qigong* works to adjust the qi activity and dredge meridians.

松胯[sōng kuà] relaxing the crotch 打太极拳必须 ~。The crotch must be relaxed when doing tai chi chuan. / ~ 有利于调整身法。Relaxing the crotch helps to adjust posture.

送 sòng

送服[sòng fú] taking medicines with liquid 酒 ~ taking medicinals with rice wine/水 ~ taking drugs with water

酥夙肃素宿 SU

酥 sū

酥油[sū yóu] butter

夙 sù

夙愿[sù yuàn] long-cherished dream

肃 sù

肃降 [sù jiàng] purifying and down-sending 肺主 ~ The lung dominates purification and down-sending of qi.

素 sù

素食 [sù shí] vegetarian food ~ 者 vegetarian

素养[sù yǎng] accomplishment 有文学 ~ being well versed in literature

素质 [sù zhì] nature; disposition 她有好教师的 ~。She has the makings of a good teacher.

宿 sù

宿疾[sù jí] chronic complaint

宿食[sù shí] retained food ~ 不化 failure to remove the retained food/ ~ 停聚, 久而成积。Diseases may develop when there is retained food in the body for days.

酸蒜算 SUAN

酸 suān

酸[suān] sour ~ 味 sour taste/喜食 ~ preference for sour taste/ ~ 走筋, 筋病无多食 ~。Sour flavor acts on tendons, so avoid sour food in patients with tendon problems.

酸甘化阴[suān gān huà yīn]yin

transformed from sour and sweet flavor 芍药、甘草相配既可缓急止痛，又可 ~。*Shaoyao* (White Peony Root) and *Gancao* (Liquorice Root) are administered together to subside spasm and pain, and at the same time to replenish yin with their sour and sweet flavor.

酸苦甘辛咸[suān kǔ gān xīn xián] sour, bitter, sweet, pungent and salty flavor

酸梅[suān méi] sweet-sour smoked plum ~汤 sweet-sour smoked plum juice

酸入肝[suān rù gān] sour flavor acting on the liver

酸枣[suān zǎo] wild jujube

蒜 suàn

蒜瓣儿[suàn bàn er] garlic clove

蒜黄[suàn huáng] blanched garlic leaf

蒜苗[suàn miáo] garlic shoot

算 suàn

算命[suàn mìng] fortune telling

随髓 SUI

随 suí

随证取穴[suí zhèng qǔ xué] acupoint selected according to patterns

髓 suí

髓海[suǐ hǎi] reservoir of marrow, brain ~空虚 hollow feeling of the brain

孙飧损 SUN

孙 sūn

孙络[sūn luò] tertiary collateral

飧 sūn

飧泄[sūn xiè] lienteric diarrhea

损 sǔn

损伤[sǔn shāng] trauma; injury

损腰[sǔn yāo] strain of the lumbar muscle

缩所锁 SUO

缩 suō

缩尿[suō niào] arresting polyuria 补肾 ~ reinforcing the kidney to arrest polyuria

所 suǒ

所食之味，与病相宜[suǒ shí zhī wèi, yǔ bìng xiāng yí] taking food that is beneficial to one's condition

锁 suǒ

锁骨[suǒ gǔ] clavicle ~骨折 clavicle fracture

S

T

踏 TA

踏 tà

踏青[tà qīng] going for a spring outing 春日～令人心情愉快。Going for a spring outing makes people enjoy ease of mind.

踏跳法[tà tiào fǎ] gentle stepping

踏雪[tà xuě] walking in the snow

踏月[tà yuè] taking a walk in the moon light

苔胎太 TAI

苔 tāi

苔[tāi] tongue coating, fur ～厚腻主热病。Thick and greasy fur suggests a febrile disease.

苔色[tāi sè] color of the tongue coating

胎 tāi

胎动不安[tāi dòng bù ān] threatened abortion

胎寒[tāi hán] fetal cold pattern

胎疾[tāi jí] disease of the newborn

胎记[tāi jì] birthmark ～多对小儿身体无妨。In general, birthmark does not do any harm to infants.

胎教音乐[tāi jiào yīn yuè] antenatal music training 在孕期常听～,于妈妈和孩子均有益。Antenatal music training is good for both the fetus and pregnant woman.

胎漏[tāi lòu] vaginal bleeding during pregnancy

胎盘[tāi pán] placenta

胎热[tāi rè] heat in newborn

胎弱[tāi ruò] congenital feebleness of fetus

胎食[tāi shí] saliva swallowing ～是古代非常倡导的一种强身方法。Saliva swallowing was an ancient approach to toning up the body. / ～为气功术语。Saliva swallowing is a term in *qigong*.

胎位不正[tāi wèi bù zhèng] abnormal position of fetus

胎息[tāi xī] fetal respiration 得～者,能不以鼻口嘘吸,如人在胞胎之中。In fetal breathing, people do not breathe with the nose or mouth, but they breathe like a fetus.

胎痫[tāi xián] neonatal convulsion

胎痣[tāi zhì] birthmark

太 tài

太冲脉[tài chōng mài] Thoroughfare Vessel ～盛,天癸至,月事以时下。When qi and blood are full in the

Thoroughfare Vessel, the sex-stimulating essence develops and the menstrual function establishes.

太饥伤脾［tài jī shāng pí］spleen injured by extreme hunger ~，太饱伤气。Extreme hunger injures the spleen and eating one's fill injures qi.

太极［tài jí］tai chi, infinite void ~ 剑 tai chi sword/ ~ 推手 hand pushing in tai chi chuan/ ~ 云手 hands moving like clouds in tai chi chuan/ ~ 生两仪, 两仪生四象, 四象生八卦。Tai chi generated the two *Yi* or symbols, which were distinguished as yin and yang. From the two *Yi* were generated the four *Xiang* or figures. By similarly combining the four *Xiang* the Eight Trigrams were produced.

太极拳［tài jí quán］tai chi chuan 二十四式 ~ 24 stylized tai chi chuan

太极图［tài jí tú］symbol of the ultimate supreme

太息［tài xī］deep sighing 肝气郁滞, 善 ~ One tends to sigh deeply when there is stagnation of liver-qi.

太虚［tài xū］the universe ~ 寥廓 vast universe

太阳病［tài yáng bìng］*Taiyang* disorder

太阳腑证［tài yáng fǔ zhèng］*Taiyang fu*-organ pattern

太阳经证［tài yáng jīng zhèng］*Taiyang* meridian pattern

太阳人［tài yáng rén］*Taiyang*-featured person

太阳中风［tài yáng zhòng fēng］attack of the *Taiyang* meridian by wind

太医［tài yī］imperial court physician ~ 院 Imperial Medical Institution

太阴病［tài yīn bìng］*Taiyin* disorder

太阴人［tài yīn rén］*Taiyin*-featured person

痰探炭 TAN
痰 tán

痰［tán］sputum, phlegm

痰火［tán huǒ］phlegm-fire ~ 头痛 headache due to phlegm-fire

痰火扰心［tán huǒ rǎo xīn］phlegm-fire agitating the heart

痰厥［tán jué］syncope due to phlegm

痰迷心窍［tán mí xīn qiào］heart fogged by phlegm ~，神昏，谵语。Heart fogged by phlegm is marked by unconsciousness and delirium.

痰热内扰［tán rè nèi rǎo］inner disturbance due to phlegm-heat

痰湿［tán shī］phlegm-dampness 温化 ~ resolving phlegm-dampness with medicinals warm in property

痰湿质［tán shī zhì］type of phlegm-dampness constitution ~ 需健脾利湿。It is advisable to invigorate the spleen to resolve dampness for people with the phlegm-dampness constitution.

痰饮［tán yǐn］retained phlegm and

morbid fluid ~ 胁痛 hypochondrial pain due to retention of phlegm and morbid fluid

痰浊阻肺［tán zhuó zǔ fèi］lung obstructed by phlegm

探 tàn

探吐［tàn tǔ］inducing vomiting

炭 tàn

炭画［tàn huà］charcoal drawing

汤唐溏糖烫 TANG

汤 tāng

汤包［tāng bāo］steamed bun stuffed with juicy meat

汤剂［tāng jì］herbal decoction ~ 的疗效迅速。Herbal decoction has a quick effect.

汤料［tāng liào］soup stock

汤面［tāng miàn］noodles in soup

汤圆［tāng yuán］round dumplings

唐 táng

唐诗宋词［táng shī sòng cí］poems of the Tang Dynasty（618-907）and rhymed verses of the Song Dynasty（960-1127）她很喜欢中国古典文学，~ 等都涉猎过。She is very fond of Chinese classical literature and has spent some time reading the poetry of the Tang and Song dynasties（618-1127）.

唐装［táng zhuāng］traditional Chinesestyle attire

溏 táng

溏便［táng biàn］loose feces 脾胃阳虚，~ 不止。Deficiency in the spleen and stomach results in excreting loose feces.

溏泄［táng xiè］sloppy diarrhea

糖 táng

糖浆剂［táng jiāng jì］syrup 止咳 ~ cough syrup

糖色［táng sè］half-burnt sugar used to color meat

烫 tàng

烫酒［tàng jiǔ］heating rice wine

烫伤［tàng shāng］scald，burn ~ 膏 ointment for scalds

桃陶 TAO

桃 táo

桃花癣［táo huā xuǎn］peach-blossom lichen

陶 táo

陶冶［táo yě］moulding ~ 情操 shaping one's values

特 TE

特 tè

特禀质［tè bǐng zhì］specific type of constitution ~ 宜益气固表，养血消风。It is advisable to reinforce qi and secure the exterior, enrich blood and subside wind for people with the specific type of constitution.

特色菜［tè sè cài］speciality 今天你们

有什么 ~? What speciality do you have today?

特效药[tè xiào yào] specific remedy 目前尚无治疗艾滋病的 ~。At present, there are no specific remedies for AIDS.

踢提体 TI

踢 tī

踢键子[tī jiàn zi] kicking shuttlecock ~对活动关节,加强韧带有良好的作用。Kicking shuttlecock is good for joints and ligaments.

踢腿[tī tuǐ] split kick

提 tí

提插[tí chā] lifting and thrusting ~补泻 reinforcing-reducing by lifting and thrusting the needle

提肛[tí gāng] lifting the anus ~法治疗便秘 lifting the anus to relieve constipation

体 tǐ

体劳勿极[tǐ láo wù jí] moderate manual labor

体弱[tǐ ruò] weak ~多病 weak and ill/~ 气虚 qi deficiency due to frail health

体育[tǐ yù] sports; physical education

体欲常劳[tǐ yù cháng láo] doing manual labour often ~,但勿过极。Do manual labour often, but never too much.

体针[tǐ zhēn] body acupuncture ~麻醉 body acupuncture anesthesia

体质[tǐ zhì] constitution 中医 ~学 theory of constitution in traditional Chinese medicine/ ~ 虚弱 having weak constitution

天添田恬甜填 TIAN

天 tiān

天地[tiān dì] universe, Heaven and Earth ~合气,人偶自生。The qi from Heaven and Earth converges to form human beings. /人以 ~ 之气生,四时之法成。Human beings come into existence as a result of the qi of Heaven and Earth in accordance with the laws of the four seasons.

天干[tiān gān] Heavenly Stems 阴历用 ~ 地支纪年。In the traditional Chinese calendar the years are designated by the Heavenly Stems and Earthly Branches.

天癸[tiān guǐ] sex-stimulating essence ~竭 exhaustion of the sex-stimulating essence/二八,肾气盛, ~ 至。At the age of sixteen kidney-qi is abundant and sex-stimulating essence develops. / ~ 与人体的生长发育及生殖有关。The sex-stimulating essence is related to human's growth, development and reproduction.

天命[tiān mìng] fate; a full natural span of life 谨道如法,长有 ~。Close abidance by such a way of

T

cultivating health will enable one to enjoy a full natural span of life.

天年[tiān nián] natural span of life 颐养 ~ taking good care of oneself so as to live out one's years to the fullest

天气[tiān qì] weather

天然食品[tiān rán shí pǐn] natural food

天然氧吧[tiān rán yǎng bā] natural oxygen bar

天然医学[tiān rán yī xué] nature medicine

天人合一[tiān rén hé yī] unity of the Heaven and humanity, holistic view of the Heaven and environment

天人相应[tiān rén xiāng yìng] correspondence between man and universe, relevant adaptation of the human body to the natural environment ~的整体观 integrated conception of correspondence between man and universe/ ~是中医基础理论重要的特点之一。Relevant adaptation of the human body to natural environment is one of the important theoretical characteristics of the basic philosophy in traditional Chinese medicine.

天时[tiān shí] timeliness ~ 地利人和 favorable timing, geographical and human conditions/养生不仅需要考虑人和, 还需要考虑 ~。In health preservation we have to consider favorable timing as well as harmony among people.

天行赤眼[tiān xíng chì yǎn] acute contagious conjunctivitis

天行温疫[tiān xíng wēn yì] epidemic disease ~ 具有传染性。Epidemic disease is infectious.

天性[tiān xìng] nature 他 ~ 爱唠叨。He goes on and on by nature. /她 ~ 善良。She is kind-hearted.

天真[tiān zhēn] simple and unaffected ~ 烂漫 innocent and artless/ ~ 无邪 innocent

添 tiān

添加剂[tiān jiā jì] additive 食品 ~ food additive

田 tián

田夫寿[tián fū shòu] a long life enjoyed by farmers ~ , 膏梁夭。Farmers usually enjoy a long life while wealthy people die young.

田园[tián yuán] fields and gardens ~ 诗 pastoral poetry

恬 tián

恬淡[tián dàn] indifferent to fame and gain ~ 寡欲 being contented and having few desires

恬淡虚无[tián dàn xū wú] indifferent to fame and gain, and devoid of distraction ~ , 真气从之。It is proper to be indifferent to fame and gain, and devoid of distraction, then healthy qi flows smoothly.

恬淡之味[tián dàn zhī wèi] insipid taste 唯 ~ , 方能补精。Medicinals with insipid taste replenish essence.

甜 tián

甜点［tián diǎn］dessert

甜酒［tián jiǔ］sweet wine

甜美［tián měi］sweet ~ 生活 happy life/味道 ~ having a sweet taste/音色 ~ having a sweet voice

甜蜜素［tián mì sù］cyclamate

甜面酱［tián miàn jiàng］sweet sauce made from fermented flour

填 tián

填精［tián jīng］replenishing essence 补肾 ~ replenishing kidney-essence/ ~ 补髓 replenishing marrow and essence

条调挑跳 TIAO

条 tiáo

条剂［tiáo jì］medicinal strip

调 tiáo

调畅气机［tiáo chàng qì jī］regulating qi activity 健脾和胃， ~ strengthening the spleen and harmonizing the stomach to regulate the qi activity

调服［tiáo fú］infusion for oral taking

调和［tiáo hé］harmonizing ~ 肝脾 harmonizing the liver and spleen/ ~ 气血 regulating qi and blood/ ~ 营卫 harmonizing the nutritive and defensive levels/逍遥散具有 ~ 肝脾的作用。 The *Xiaoyao* Powder is applicable to harmonizing the liver and spleen.

调和诸药［tiáo hé zhū yào］coordinating the action of various ingredients in a formula 使药甘草,多具有 ~ 的作用。 *Gancao*（Licorice Root）, serving as a guide medicinal may coordinate the action of other ingredients in a formula.

调和诸脏［tiáo hé zhū zàng］regulating the function of the *zang*-organs ~ 是中医治疗内伤病的一个重要原则。 Regulating the function of various *zang*-organs is an important principle to relieve the internal injury in traditional Chinese medicine.

调经［tiáo jīng］regulating menstruation

调理［tiáo lǐ］nursing one's health; regulating 综合 ~ comprehensive nurse of one's health

调气［tiáo qì］regulating qi ~ 疏肝法 regulating qi flow and soothing the liver/ ~ 止痛 regulating qi flow to kill pain/ ~ 解郁 regulating qi flow and relieving stagnancy

调摄［tiáo shè］fine-tuning 心理 ~ adjusting one's psychology/ ~ 情志 adjusting emotions

调身［tiáo shēn］posture management ~ 养性 posture management and cultivation of oneself/ ~ 要领 essentials of posture management

调神［tiáo shén］regulating mental activities ~ 养生 health preservation by regulating mental activities

调息［tiáo xī］regulating breathing

调心［tiáo xīn］training of the mind ~ 安神 training and calming the mind

调养［tiáo yǎng］taking good care of

oneself; being nursed back to health
身体 ~ building up one's health

调整阴阳 [tiáo zhěng yīn yáng]
regulating yin and yang

挑 tiǎo
挑治 [tiǎo zhì] piercing method

跳 tiào
跳大神 [tiào dà shén] sorcerer's dance
in a trance
跳绳 [tiào shéng] rope skipping
跳跃运动 [tiào yuè yùn dòng] jumping
jack

铁 TIE
铁 tiě
铁裆功 [tiě dāng gōng] iron crotch
exercise ~ 治疗阳痿。The iron crotch
exercise treats impotence.

亭庭挺 TING
亭 tíng
亭亭玉立 [tíng tíng yù lì] slim and
graceful

庭 tíng
庭院 [tíng yuàn] front courtyard

挺 tǐng
挺胸拔背 [tǐng xiōng bá bèi]
straightening up, holding one's body
erect ~ 是形体健美操的基本要求。
Straightening up and holding one's
body erect are the basic requirement
of the aerobic exercise.

通同铜童痛 TONG
通 tōng
通风 [tōng fēng] ventilating 不 ~ poorly
ventilated/ ~ 即阖。Shut the windows
when wind is blowing.

通剂 [tōng jì] obstruction-removing
formula

通利 [tōng lì] easing ~ 关节 easing the
tension of joints/邪阻经络, 气血运
行不畅, 治宜 ~ 关节。It is advisable
to ease the tension of joints caused by
impeded flow of qi and blood due to
retention of pathogenic factors in
meridians. / ~ 血脉 promoting blood
circulation

通乳 [tōng rǔ] promoting lactation ~ 药
lactation-promoting medicines

通下 [tōng xià] laxative remedy

通阳 [tōng yáng] activating yang ~ 利水
activating yang for diuresis/ ~ 散结
activating yang to disintegrate masses

通因通用 [tōng yīn tōng yòng] using
purgatives to treat diarrhea

同 tóng
同病异食 [tóng bìng yì shí] different
diets for patients with the same
disease ~ 是饮食疗法的一大基本原
则。Different diets for patients with
the same disease is an important rule
in dietotherapy.

同病异治 [tóng bìng yì zhì] treating the
same disease with different methods

同身寸 [tóng shēn cùn] proportional

body-*cun* 拇指 ~ measurement with the proportional thumb body-*cun*/中指 ~ measurement with the proportional middle finger body-*cun*

铜 tóng

铜人[tóng rén] bronze figure 针灸 ~ acupuncture bronze figure

童 tóng

童男[tóng nán] virgin boy

童女[tóng nǚ] virgin maid

童声[tóng shēng] child's voice ~ 合唱 children's chorus

童心[tóng xīn] childlike innocence ~ 未泯 still preserving traces of childlike innocence

童颜鹤发[tóng yán hè fà] having white hair and ruddy complexion

童真[tóng zhēn] naivety 充满 ~ 的感情 full of childlike simplicity

童子鸡[tóng zǐ jī] young chicken

童子劳[tóng zǐ láo] child consumptive disease

痛 tòng

痛[tòng] pain 关节 ~ joint pain/心绞 ~ angina pectoris/ ~ 无定处 pain of unfixed location

痛痹[tòng bì] arthralgia due to cold

痛风[tòng fēng] gout

痛经[tòng jīng] dysmenorrhea

头透 TOU

头 tóu

头发稀疏[tóu fà xī shū] thinning hair

头汗[tóu hàn] sweating from the head

头皮瘙痒[tóu pí sāo yǎng] scalp itching

头皮针[tóu pí zhēn] scalp acupuncture ~ 疗法 scalp acupuncture therapy/ ~ 治疗高血压疗效确切。Scalp acupuncture is most effective against hypertension.

头如顶物[tóu rú dǐng wù] keeping the head upright as if something is on its top

头痛[tóu tòng] headache

头晕[tóu yūn] dizziness

头胀[tóu zhàng] distending feeling in the head

头正[tóu zhèng] keeping the head upright

头重[tóu zhòng] heaviness feeling in the head ~ 脚轻 heavy head and light feet accompanied by unsteady gaits

透 tòu

透刺[tòu cì] penetrative needling

透关射甲[tòu guān shè jiǎ] superficial veins extending throughout the three passes towards the index finger tip ~ 属病危。When the superficial veins extend throughout the three passes towards the index finger tip, it is a critical condition.

透汗[tòu hàn] breaking out in a sweat 一身 ~ sweat all over

透气通风[tòu qì tōng fēng] air 他有点头晕,请开窗 ~。He is a bit dizzy, please open the windows and let in some fresh air.

透视[tòu shì] clairvoyance 具有～功能的人 clairvoyant

透邪[tòu xié] expelling pathogens

土吐吐 TU

土 tǔ

土特产[tǔ tè chǎn] local speciality

土形人[tǔ xíng rén] earth-featured person ～主要病在水行,包括肾、膀胱、骨和腰腿等。Earth-featured people often suffer from disorders of the water phase (kidney) manifested itself as problems of the kidney, urinary bladder, bone, lower back and leg.

吐 tǔ

吐故纳新[tǔ gù nà xīn] getting rid of the stale and taking in the fresh

吐纳[tǔ nà] expiration and inspiration ～调息 regulating expiration and inspiration/～养生法 keeping fit through expiration and inspiration exercises

吐弄舌[tǔ nòng shé] protruding and waggling of the tongue

吐 tù

吐法[tù fǎ] emetic therapy

吐蛔[tù huí] vomiting of ascaris

吐剂[tù jì] emetic 催～emetic

吐血[tù xiě] hematemesis

推腿退 TUI

推 tuī

推陈出新[tuī chén chū xīn] weeding out the old to bring forth the new

推法[tuī fǎ] pushing

推罐法[tuī guàn fǎ] mobile cupping

推磨法[tuī mò fǎ] stroking

推拿[tuī ná] *tuina*-massage ～师 *tuina*-massage therapist

推寻[tuī xún] pushing and searching

腿 tuǐ

腿功[tuǐ gōng] leg training

退 tuì

退针[tuì zhēn] needle withdrawing

吞 TUN

吞 tūn

吞食梗塞[tūn shí gěng sè] difficulty of swallowing

脱唾 TUO

脱 tuō

脱发[tuō fà] hair loss 遗传性～hereditary hair loss

脱肛[tuō gāng] prolapse of the rectum

脱位[tuō wèi] dislocation 掌指关节～dislocation of the phalangeal joint of hand

脱阳[tuō yáng] yang depletion

脱脂奶粉[tuō zhī nǎi fěn] non-fat milk powder

唾 tuò

唾[tuò] saliva;spittle ～血 spitting blood

W

歪喝外 WAI

歪 wāi

歪斜舌[wāi xié shé] deviated tongue

喝 wāi

喝僻不遂[wāi pì bù suí] facial paralysis and hemiplegia after stroke

外 wài

外风[wài fēng] external wind ～致病可见恶寒、微发热等。Diseases due to external wind are marked by chills, mild fever, etc.

外感 [wài gǎn] external contraction, disease or morbid condition produced by any of the six excesses or other noxious factors ～六淫邪气 contraction of the six excesses/风寒 ～则表现为恶寒发热身痛。Contraction of wind-cold manifests itself as aversion to cold, fever and general pain.

外功[wài gōng] dynamic *qigong*

外廉[wài lián] lateral aspect ～疮 ulcer at the lateral tibia

外气[wài qì] emitted qi

外伤[wài shāng] traumatic injury ～性骨折 traumatic fracture

外肾[wài shèn] testis

外因[wài yīn] external cause ～致病 disease due to the external cause/ ～：外感六淫,"起于经络,合于脏腑"。The external causes are the externally contracted six excesses that "first attack the meridians and then affect the *zang-fu* organs".

外御内守[wài yù nèi shǒu] preventing attack from outside and guarding internally

外治[wài zhì] external treatment 疡疮疖肿等外科疾病,多采取 ～法。External treatment is used for external afflictions such as abscesses and boils.

弯丸玩顽挽晚脘万 WAN

弯 wān

弯针[wān zhēn] bending of a needle 在针刺过程中导致 ～的原因很多。There are several reasons leading to bending of a needle in the course of acupuncture treatment.

丸 wán

丸剂[wán jì] pill; bolus 蜜 ～ honeyed bolus/水 ～ watered pill/ ～是中医治病常用的一种剂型。Pills or boluses are the frequently-used drug forms in

W

traditional Chinese therapy.

丸子[wán zi] ball 肉 ~ meat ball

玩 wán

玩赏[wán shǎng] enjoying

顽 wán

顽痰[wán tán] obstinate phlegm ~ 为患,易变生他病。 Suffering from obstinate phlegm tends to cause other diseases.

顽症[wán zhèng] chronic and stubborn disease

挽 wǎn

挽耳[wǎn ěr] pulling ears ~ 是一种古代健身法。 Ear pulling was an ancient approach to keeping fit.

晚 wǎn

晚秋[wǎn qiū] late autumn

脘 wǎn

脘痞[wǎn pǐ] gastric stuffiness

脘痛[wǎn tòng] stomachache

万 wàn

万物[wàn wù] everything on earth ~ 悉备 creation of all things on earth/ ~ 以荣。 All things are flourishing on earth. / ~ 资始 origin of all things on earth/天下 ~ 生于有, 有生于无。 Everything on earth is formed by something, and something is generated by nothing.

亡妄望 WANG

亡 wáng

亡血家[wáng xuè jiā] patient suffering from hemorrhagic diseases ~ ,不可发汗。 For patients suffering from hemorrhagic diseases it is forbidden to induce sweating.

亡阳[wáng yáng] yang depletion 多汗 ~ profuse sweating leading to depletion of yang

亡阴[wáng yīn] yin depletion ~ 常见身体干瘦,皮肤皱褶,烦躁,昏迷谵语等。 Depletion of yin is often characterized by emaciation, wrinkled skin, restlessness, coma and delibrium.

妄 wàng

妄念[wàng niàn] wild idea, improper thought 挥之不去的 ~ difficult to wipe away wild ideas/消除 ~ discarding improper thoughts

妄听[wàng tīng] improper hearing 耳 ~ 则惑 improper hearing leading to confusion

妄言[wàng yán] talking nonsense; wild talk 一者不 ~ 。 First do not talk nonsense.

望 wàng

望面色[wàng miàn sè] inspection of the complexion

望舌[wàng shé] inspection of the tongue

望神[wàng shén] inspection of vitality ~ 是判断病情的一种方法。 Inspection of vitality is a way to determine the condition of a disease.

望形态[wàng xíng tài] inspection of the bodily figure and behavior

望诊[wàng zhěn] inspection, looking

望指纹[wàng zhǐ wén]inspection of the superficial venule of the index finger in infants

煨微维围伪萎痿未胃畏卫 WEI

煨 wēi

煨[wēi] roasting in ashes 葱蒜 ~ roasting with Chinese onion and garlic/姜 ~ roasted ginger/酒 ~ roasting with rice wine in ashes

微 wēi

微波针灸疗法[wēi bō zhēn jiǔ liáo fǎ] microwave acupuncture therapy

微脉[wēi mài]faint pulse

微热[wēi rè]low fever

微针系统[wēi zhēn xì tǒng] microsystem acupuncture

维 wéi

维医学[wéi yī xué]Uighur medicine

围 wéi

围棋[wéi qí] Go 下 ~ playing a game of Go

伪 wěi

伪品[wěi pǐn]adulterant

萎 wěi

萎靡[wěi mí] dispirited ~ 不振 in low spirits

痿 wěi

痿软舌[wěi ruǎn shé]flaccid tongue

痿证[wěi zhèng]flaccidity of limbs

未 wèi

未病先防[wèi bìng xiān fáng] prevention first (before onset of disease) ~是预防 医学的核心。Prevention first is the key of preventive medicine.

胃 wèi

胃[wèi] stomach ~ 寒 cold in the stomach

胃不和[wèi bù hé] stomach disorder ~ 则卧不安。Stomach disorder disturbs sleep.

胃肠病[wèi cháng bìng] gastric and intestinal disorder

胃家实[wèi jiā shí]excess pattern of the stomach and intestine with dryness-heat

胃经[wèi jīng] Stomach Meridian

胃气[wèi qì] stomach-qi ~ 虚 deficiency of stomach-qi/ ~ 不和 disorder of stomach-qi/ ~ 上逆 upward attack by stomach-qi/ ~ 衰败 exhaustion of stomach-qi

胃热[wèi rè]stomach-heat ~ 则消谷善 饥 stomach-heat leading to abnormally increased appetite with frequent hunger

胃脘[wèi wǎn] stomach ~ 冷痛 cold pain in the stomach / ~ 痞闷 stuffiness in the stomach

胃之大络[wèi zhī dà luò]large stomach collateral

胃主腐熟[wèi zhǔ fǔ shú] stomach performing the function of decomposing food stuff

胃主受纳[wèi zhǔ shòu nà] stomach performing the function of receiving food

畏 wèi

畏光[wèi guāng]photophobia

畏寒[wèi hán]aversion to cold 阳虚病人多见～肢冷。Aversion to cold and cold limbs are often seen in patients with deficiency of yang.

卫 wèi

卫分证[wèi fèn zhèng]disorder of the defensive level

卫气[wèi qì]defensive qi ～不行 failure of defensive qi to move/～不固 insecurity of defensive qi/～不固, 则易致表虚证。Insecurity of defensive qi brings about an exterior deficiency pattern.

卫气营血辨证[wèi qì yíng xuè biàn zhèng]differentiation of patterns by analysis of the conditions of the defensive, qi, nutritive and blood levels

温瘟闻文问 WEN

温 wēn

温病[wēn bìng]warm-pathogen disease ～的预后, 多以胃气的有无为标准, 有一份胃气, 便有一份生机。A favorable or unfavorable prognosis of a warm-pathogen disease depends on existence or absence of stomach-qi. There is stomach-qi, there is a chance of survival. /～后期, 上损及下。At the late stage of a warm-pathogen disease the upper impairment involves the lower part of the body.

温补[wēn bǔ]tonifying with medicinals warm in property ～脾胃 reinforcing the spleen and stomach with medicinals warm in property/～肾阳 strengthening kidney-yang with medicinals warm in nature /羊肉、大枣、冬瓜等常作为冬令～的食物。Lamb, Chinese date and wax gourd are food of warm nature serving as winter tonics.

温法[wēn fǎ]warming therapy 里寒实证或虚寒证, 宜选用～。The warming therapy is adopted for an excess pattern of interior cold or a deficiency cold pattern.

温服[wēn fú]taking herbal decoction warm 汤药一般多宜～。In general hebal decoctions are taken warm.

温和灸[wēn hé jiǔ]mild moxibustion

温化寒痰[wēn huà hán tán]resolving cold-phlegm with medicinals warm in property 寒痰证用～法治疗。A cold-phlegm pattern is resolved with medicinals warm in property.

温经散寒[wēn jīng sàn hán]warming meridians to dissipate cold

温里[wēn lǐ]warming the interior ～散寒 warming the interior to dissipate cold/里寒证用～法治疗。Warming the interior is adopted to treat an interior cold pattern.

温暖[wēn nuǎn]warm 阳光～warm sunshine

温脾[wēn pí]warming the spleen 脾寒

证用～法治疗。A spleen-cold pattern is treated by warming the spleen.

温泉浴[wēn quán yù] hot-spring bath

温热[wēn rè] warm-heat

温肾[wēn shèn] warming the kidney ～壮阳 warming the kidney and invigorating yang

温水送服[wēn shuǐ sòng fú] taken with warm water

温胃[wēn wèi] warming the stomach 寒邪犯胃或胃阳虚证,用～建中法治疗。Warming the stomach to strengthen its function is for invasion of the stomach by cold or deficiency of stomach-yang.

温下[wēn xià] purgation with medicinals warm in property 寒积便秘选用～法。Purgative medicinals warm in property to cause bowel movements are prescribed for constipation due to retained cold.

温邪[wēn xié] warm-pathogen ～上受,首先犯肺,逆传心包。Warm pathogen first invades the lung, and then the pericardium.

温馨[wēn xīn] cosy

温性[wēn xìng] warm in property ～药物 medicinals warm in property/辛～药物,易伤人体正气。Medicinals pungent in flavor and warm in property are prone to impair healthy qi. / ～是药物四气之一。Warm property is one of the four properties of herbal medicinals.

温阳[wēn yáng] warming and activating yang ～利水 warming and activating yang for diuresis/ ～散寒 warming and activating yang to dissipate cold

温针灸[wēn zhēn jiǔ] acupuncture with mild moxibustion ～是针刺与艾灸结合应用的一种方法。Acupuncture with mild moxibustion is one that combines acupuncture with moxibustion.

温中[wēn zhōng] warming the middle-energizer ～降气 warming the middle-energizer to bring down the rebellious qi/ ～行气 warming the middle-energizer to promote qi flow

温中补虚[wēn zhōng bǔ xū] warming the middle-energizer and tonifying in a deficiency condition

温中止呕[wēn zhōng zhǐ ǒu] warming the middle-energizer to check vomiting ～法治疗脾胃中焦虚寒之呕吐。Warming the middle-energizer to check vomiting is a way to relieve vomiting due to deficiency and cold in the spleen and stomach.

温中止痛[wēn zhōng zhǐ tòng] warming the middle-energizer to kill pain 脾胃虚寒,腹部隐隐作痛,治宜～,散寒和胃。Warming the middle- energizer to kill pain is adopted to dissipate cold from the spleen and stomach in a deficiency condition, and stop abdominal dull pain.

瘟 wēn

瘟毒［wēn dú］pestilent toxin ~ 发斑 pestilent maculae

瘟痧［wēn shā］epidemic eruptive disease

瘟疫［wēn yì］pestilence 防止 ~ 蔓延 preventing the spread of pestilence/ ~ 流行地区 pestilence-ridden area

闻 wén

闻气味［wén qì wèi］smelling odor

闻声音［wén shēng yīn］listening to voice

闻诊［wén zhěn］listening and smelling

文 wén

文火［wén huǒ］lower flame ~ 煎 simmering/煎药, 温补之剂多用 ~ 。Decocting herbal mdicinals with warm and tonifying nature needs lower flame. /煎药煮沸后, 用 ~ 继续煎煮。After boiling the herbal ingredients are continuously simmered.

文静［wén jìng］gentle and quiet

文眉［wén méi］tattooing the eyebrows

文身［wén shēn］tattoo; tattooing ~ 师 tattooist/他的背上有一个龙 ~ 图案。His back was tattooed with a dragon.

问 wèn

问诊［wèn zhěn］asking

卧 WO

卧 wò

卧如弓［wò rú gōng］sleeping bent like an arch ~ , 有利于人体放松全身。An arch sleeping pose is more relaxing.

卧式［wò shì］lying posture 半 ~ semi-recumbent posture/侧 ~ lateral recumbent posture/仰 ~ supine posture

卧须闭口［wò xū bì kǒu］keeping the mouth closed in sleep ~ 则元气不出, 邪气不入。Keeping the mouth closed in sleep can help preserve healthy qi and prevent pathogenic factors from invasion.

乌巫屋无五午武物寤悟误恶 WU

乌 wū

乌痧［wū shā］purplish eruption ~ 惊风 infantile convulsion with cyanosis

乌须发［wū xū fà］blackening the beard and hair

巫 wū

巫医［wū yī］witch doctor

屋 wū

屋漏脉［wū lòu mài］roof-leaking pulse

无 wú

无瘢痕灸［wú bān hén jiǔ］non-scarring moxibustion

无病早防［wú bìng zǎo fáng］prevention first

无毒治病十去其九［wú dú zhì bìng shí qù qí jiǔ］When more neutral medicinals are used, they should be discontinued when nine-tenths of the pathogen is eliminated.

无伐天和［wú fá tiān hé］avoiding violation of natural harmony

无饥无饱［wú jī wú bǎo］not eating too much or too little 凡食之道，～。 When one has a meal, he should not eat too much or too little.

无名肿毒［wú míng zhǒng dú］undefined swelling and sore

无头疽［wú tóu jū］deep cellulitis

无为［wú wéi］acting by not acting

无厌于日［wú yàn yú rì］no detestation of long and hot day

五 wǔ

五菜为充［wǔ cài wéi chōng］five kinds of vegetables as complement

五迟五软［wǔ chí wǔ ruǎn］five kinds of retardation and flaccidity in infants

五刺［wǔ cì］five acupuncture techniques

五畜为益［wǔ chù wéi yì］five types of meat as tonic

五更泻［wǔ gēng xiè］dawn diarrhea

五谷为养［wǔ gǔ wéi yǎng］five kinds of grains as staple food to nourish the body

五官［wǔ guān］five sense organs

五果为助［wǔ guǒ wéi zhù］five kinds of fruits as supplement nutrition

五戒［wǔ jiè］Bodhidharma's five commandments against killing, stealing, obscenity, telling lies and drinking liquor

五劳［wǔ láo］five kinds of strain ～所伤 impairment from the five kinds of strain

五气［wǔ qì］five kinds of qi 天食人以～。Heaven nourishes humans with five kinds of qi.

五禽戏［wǔ qín xì］Five Mimic-animal Frolics ～为三国时期华佗所创的一种保健操。The Five Mimic-animal Frolics is a fit-keeping exercise designed by Hua Tuo in the period of the Three Kingdoms (220-280).

五色［wǔ sè］five colors: dark greyish green, yellow, red, white and black

五十肩［wǔ shí jiān］periarthritis of the shoulder

五体［wǔ tǐ］five body structures

五味［wǔ wèi］five flavors: sweet, sour, bitter, pungent and salty ～偏嗜 food preference/～所禁 abstinence from the five flavors/地食人以～。Earth provides humans with five flavors.

五味所和［wǔ wèi suǒ hé］harmony between flavor and the zang-organs ～，方可健康长寿。When flavor matches with the zang-organs, one may enjoy good health and longevity.

五味所入［wǔ wèi suǒ rù］attribution of the five flavors

五心［wǔ xīn］palms, soles and chest ～烦热 a hot sensation in the palms soles and chest

五行［wǔ xíng］five phases, five elements ～相乘 over-acting among the five phases/～相克 sequential

W

restraining among the five phases/ ~
相生 sequential generating among the
five phases/ ~ 相侮 mutual counter-
restricting among the five phases

五言诗[wǔ yán shī] ancient poem with
five characters to each line

五液[wǔ yè] five kinds of secretions

五音 [wǔ yīn] five notes of the
pentatonic scale ~ 不全 singing out of
tune/ ~ 疗法 therapy with the five
notes of the pentatonic scale

五欲[wǔ yù] five desires

五脏[wǔ zàng] five zang-organs ~ 所藏
what the five zang-organs store/ ~ 所
恶 what the five zang-organs dislike/
~ 所主 what the five zang-organs
control/ ~ 藏精气而不泻。The five
zang-organs store essence without
discharge.

五脏六腑 [wǔ zàng liù fǔ] five zang
and six fu organs ~ 之精皆上注于
目。The essence of the five zang and
six fu organs ascends to the eyes.

五脏为本,杂合以养[wǔ zàng wéi běn,
zá hé yǐ yǎng] The five zang-organs
are the key element in health
preservation.

五志 [wǔ zhì] five emotional
manifestations ~ 过极 extreme
excitation of the five kinds of
emotion/ ~ 化火 fire triggered by the
five kinds of emotional excitement

午 wǔ

午后不食[wǔ hòu bù shí] not eating
food after noon

午后潮热[wǔ hòu cháo rè] afternoon
fever ~ 阴虚发热的主症为 ~ 。
Afternoon fever is the chief symptom
of fever due to yin deficiency.

武 wǔ

武火[wǔ huǒ] high flame 中药需要 ~
煮沸,然后转为小火。Decocting
herbal medicinals should use high
flame first to boil, then lower flame
follows.

物 wù

物我两忘[wù wǒ liǎng wàng] forgetting
both oneself and the external world

寤 wù

寤寐[wù mèi] asleep or awake

悟 wù

悟性[wù xìng] power of understanding

误 wù

误下[wù xià] incorrect administration of
purgatives

误诊[wù zhěn] misdiagnosis

误治[wù zhì] erroneous treatment

恶 wù

恶风[wù fēng] aversion to wind

恶寒[wù hán] aversion to cold ~ 发热
averson to cold with fever

W

X

夕稀吸息溪膝习洗喜细 XI

夕 xī

夕加［xī jiā］disease worsen in the evening

稀 xī

稀饭［xī fàn］rice or millet gruel

吸 xī

吸杯法［xī bēi fǎ］cupping

吸入法［xī rù fǎ］inhalation

息 xī

息粗［xī cū］breathing nosily

息风［xī fēng］subsiding internal wind ~ 止痉 subsiding internal wind to abate convulsion

息微［xī wēi］feeble breathing 阳气衰竭可出现 ~。Feeble breathing may be caused by exhaustion of yang-qi.

溪 xī

溪毒［xī dú］stream polluted by blood flukes

膝 xī

膝［xī］knee ~ 痛 painful knees

膝顶法［xī dǐng fǎ］knee-pushing reduction

习 xí

习俗［xí sú］custom 民间 ~ folk custom/传统 ~ traditional customs/ ~ 养生 following customs for health preservation

洗 xǐ

洗漱［xǐ shù］washing face and rinsing mouth

喜 xǐ

喜［xǐ］joy ~ 伤心 heart impaired by over-joy/ ~ 则气缓。Over-joy leads to sluggishness of heart-qi.

喜按［xǐ àn］preference for pressing

喜怒哀乐［xǐ nù āi lè］all human emotions

细 xì

细嚼慢咽［xì jiáo màn yàn］chewing thoroughly and swallowing slowly ~ 有助于消化和吸收。Chewing thoroughly and swallowing slowly when having meals help digestion and absorption.

细脉［xì mài］thready pulse 血虚多见 ~。Thready pulse is often seen in a blood deficiency case.

虾下夏 XIA

虾 xiā

虾酱［xiā jiàng］shrimp paste

虾游脉［xiā yóu mài］shrimp-darting

pulse

虾子[xiā zǐ] shrimp roe

下 xià

下按式[xià àn shì] downward pressing posture

下病上取[xià bìng shàng qǔ] treating diseases in the lower part of the body by needling applied to the upper

下法[xià fǎ] purgation

下工[xià gōng] unqualified physician in ancient times ~ 守其已成,因败其形。Unqualified physicians do not understand the importance of early prevention and resort to treatment only when the disease has already emerged.

下合穴[xià hé xué] lower He-sea acupoint

下焦[xià jiāo] lower-energizer ~ 不固 insecurity of the lower-energizer/ ~ 如渎 lower-energizer acting as a gutter

下酒[xià jiǔ] going with wine ~ 菜 dish to go with wine

下利[xià lì] diarrhea ~ 清谷 diarrhea with undigested particles

下品[xià pǐn] lower grade

下迫[xià pò] urgent desire for defecation

下棋[xiá qí] playing chess

下窍[xià qiào] lower orifices: genitals and anus

下乳[xià rǔ] promoting lactation 产后 ~ promoting lactation after childbirth

下水[xià shuǐ] offal 羊 ~ sheep offal

下元亏损[xià yuán kuī sǔn] loss of kidney-yin

夏 xià

夏道尊命[xià dào zūn mìng] fate honored by the people of the Xia Dynasty (c. 21st-c. 16th B. C.) ~ , 殷人尊神,周人尊礼法。People of the Xia Dynasty (c. 21st-c. 16th B. C.) honored fate. People of the Shang Dynasty (c. 16st-c. 11th B. C.) honored god and people of the Zhou Dynasty (c. 11th-256 B. C.) honored law and discipline.

夏防暑热[xià fáng shǔ rè] prevention of summer-heat

夏洪[xià hóng] pulse surging in summer 四季脉为春弦, ~ ,秋毛,冬石。The normal pulse conditions found in four seasons are somewhat wiry in spring, surging in summer, floating in autumn and deep in winter.

夏应中矩[xià yìng zhòng jǔ] normal surging pulse in summer ~ 为脉应气候炎热之象。Surging pulse seen in summer is normal, for it corresponds with the hot weather.

夏至[xià zhì] Summer Solstice

先鲜闲痫弦咸限线 XIAN

先 xiān

先别阴阳[xiān bié yīn yáng] distinguishing yin and yang first 善诊者,察色按脉, ~ 。An experienced

X

practitioner always distinguishes yin and yang first, then observes the complexion and takes pulse.

先春养阳[xiān chūn yǎng yáng] nourishing yang in early spring

先攻后补[xiān gōng hòu bǔ] eliminating before tonifying

先煎[xiān jiān] decocted first 矿石类药物宜~。Mineral medicinal substances should be decocted first.

先秋养阴[xiān qiū yǎng yīn] nourishing yin in early autumn

先天[xiān tiān] innate ability ~之火 innate fire/ ~之精 innate essence/肾为~之本。The kidney is the root of the innate ability.

先兆[xiān zhào] aura ~症状 precursory symptoms

鲜 xiān

鲜美[xiān měi] delicious; tasty

鲜用[xiān yòng] fresh herbs given 芦根宜~。Lugen (Reed Rhizome) is usually administrated fresh.

闲 xián

闲情逸致[xián qíng yì zhì] leisurely and carefree mood

痫 xián

痫病[xián bìng] epilepsy

弦 xián

弦[xián] string or chord of a musical instrument ~乐 stringed instrument music/ ~乐团 string orchestra

弦脉[xián mài] wiry pulse, taut pulse

沉~ deep and wiry pulse

咸 xián

咸[xián] salty flavor ~寒增液 body fluids increased by herbs salty in flavor and cold in property/ ~走血，血病无多食~。Salty flavor acts on blood, so take less salt for patients with blood disorder.

限 xiàn

限酒[xiàn jiǔ] limiting alcohol drinking

线 xiàn

线香[xiàn xiāng] joss stick ~香型 fragrance type of joss stick

相香享项相象 XIANG

相 xiāng

相伴[xiāng bàn] keeping each other company ~一生 keeping each other company whole life

相反[xiāng fǎn] incompatibility 乌头与半夏~。Wutou (Common Monkshood Mother Root) is incompatible with Banxia (Pinellia Tuber).

相杀[xiāng shā] mutual suppression

相使[xiāng shǐ] mutual assistance 款冬花配杏仁有~之用。Kuandonghua (Common Coltsfoot Flower) strengthens the effect of apricot when they are given together.

相恶[xiāng wù] mutual antagonism 生姜与黄芩 ~。Fresh ginger antagonizes the action of Huangqin (Baical Skullcap Root).

X

相须[xiāng xū] mutual accentuation

香 xiāng

香粉[xiāng fěn] cosmetic powder

香酒[xiāng jiǔ] cordiale, aromatic wine 酿制 ~ brewing cordiale/甲骨文有酿制 ~ 的记载。There are records about brewing cordiale written on the animal bones and tortoise shells.

香料[xiāng liào] spice

香囊[xiāng náng] perfume pouch, sachet bag

香甜[xiāng tián] fragrant and sweet

享 xiǎng

享年[xiǎng nián] living to the age of ~ 80 岁 passed away at the age of 80

项 xiàng

项[xiàng] nape ~ 拘急 contracture of the nape

项强[xiàng jiàng] neck rigidity

项软[xiàng ruǎn] neck flaccidity

相 xiàng

相火[xiàng huǒ] ministerial fire ~ 妄动 hyperactivity of the ministerial fire/ ~ 妄动可致遗精早泄。Hyperactivity of the ministerial fire may lead to seminal emission and premature ejaculation.

象 xiàng

象棋[xiàng qí] Chinese chess ~ 棋盘 Chinese chessboard/国际 ~ chess

消小笑哮 XIAO

消 xiāo

消导[xiāo dǎo] promoting digestion to relieve food retention ~ 药 medicinals for whetting appetite and digestion

消法[xiāo fǎ] expelling method ~ 用于消食化滞。The expelling method is used to promote digestion.

消谷善饥[xiāo gǔ shàn jī] abnormally increased appetite with frequent hunger 中消则 ~。Wasting-thirst disorder with the middle-energizer involved is marked by abnormally increased appetite with frequent hunger.

消积[xiāo jī] expelling retained food; removing stagnated qi ~ 除胀 removing food retention and distension

消积杀虫[xiāo jī shā chóng] expelling retained food and intestinal parasites

消食[xiāo shí] promoting digestion ~ 下气 promoting digestion and removing distension/山楂可以 ~ 。Hawthorn can promote digestion.

消暑[xiāo shǔ] eliminating summer-heat

消痰[xiāo tán] reducing phlegm ~ 平喘 reducing phlegm and abating panting

消炎[xiāo yán] counteracting inflammation ~ 药 anti-inflammatory agents/ ~ 疗法 antiphlogistic treatment

消痈[xiāo yōng] expelling carbuncle ~ 肿 subsidence of a carbuncle

消肿[xiāo zhǒng] subsidence of swelling ~ 解毒 subsiding a swelling and removing toxic substances/ ~ 散结 subsidence of a swelling and hard lump

小 xiǎo

小便短赤[xiǎo biàn duǎn chì] concen-

X

trated urine

小便清长[xiǎo biàn qīng cháng] long voiding of clear urine

小便失禁[xiǎo biàn shī jìn] incontinence of urine

小菜[xiǎo cài] side dish

小产[xiǎo chǎn] miscarriage

小肠经[xiǎo cháng jīng] Small Intestine Meridian

小肠气[xiǎo cháng qì] hernia

小肠实热[xiǎo cháng shí rè] excessive heat in the small intestine

小肠主液[xiǎo cháng zhǔ yè] fluid ruled by the small intestine

小炒[xiǎo chǎo] individually-cooked dish

小吃[xiǎo chī] snack

小毒治病十去其八[xiǎo dú zhì bìng shí qù qí bā] If medicinalss with mild action are used in treatment for disease, they should be discontinued when eight-tenths of the pathogen is eliminated.

小儿[xiǎo ér] child; infant, baby ～多涎 infantile dribbling/～劄目 incessant blinking in children/～客忤 child convulsive seizure due to terror

小儿推拿[xiǎo ér tuī ná] infantile *tuina*-massage

小方[xiǎo fāng] minor formula ～科 pediatrics

小腹[xiǎo fù] lower abdomen ～胀痛 distending pain in the lower abdomen

小寒[xiǎo hán] Small Cold

小夹板[xiǎo jiā bǎn] small splint

小满[xiǎo mǎn] Grain Full

小米枕[xiǎo mǐ zhěn] pillow filled with millet

小舌头[xiǎo shé tou] uvula

小暑[xiǎo shǔ] Small Heat

小雪[xiǎo xuě] Small Snow

小周天[xiǎo zhōu tiān] micro-cosmic orbit, small heavenly circuit 打通～ dredging the micro-cosmic orbit/打通～是练精化气的过程。Dredging the micro-cosmic orbit is a process to reinforce the innate essence and transform it into qi.

笑 xiào

笑口常开[xiào kǒu cháng kāi] wearing a smile often ～，青春常在。Wear a smile often, and always feel young.

哮 xiào

哮[xiào] wheezing/～为一种肺系疾病。Wheezing is a kind of lung disorder.

哮喘[xiào chuǎn] asthma 她有～病。She suffers from asthma.

哮鸣音[xiào míng yīn] wheezing

协邪胁斜泻泄 XIE

协 xié

协调阴阳[xié tiáo yīn yáng] regulating yin and yang

邪 xié

邪气[xié qì] pathogenic factor, pathogen ～入则病作。Invasion by

X

pathogenic factors brings on diseases.

邪气盛则实[xié qì shèng zé shí] An excess pattern occurs when there exist excessive pathogenic factors.

邪盛正衰[xié shèng zhèng shuāi] excessive pathogenic factors and declined healthy qi

邪正交争[xié zhèng jiāo zhēng] combat between pathogenic factors and healthy qi

邪之所凑，其气必虚[xié zhī suǒ còu, qí qì bì xū] Intrusion of pathogenic factors certainly results from insufficiency of healthy qi.

胁 xié

胁[xié] hypochondrium ~ 满 fullness in the hypochondrium/ ~ 胀 hypochondrial distension

胁下痞硬[xié xià pǐ yìng] fullness and hardness in the hypochondrium

斜 xié

斜刺[xié cì] oblique needling

斜飞脉[xié fēi mài] oblique-running pulse

斜眼[xié yǎn] strabismus, squint 中风可出现 ~ 。 Strabismus may be seen in a stroke case.

泻 xiè

泻[xiè] diarrhea

泻法[xiè fǎ] purgation; reducing method in acupuncture 推拿 ~ 是适用于下焦实证的一种治法。 The reducing maneuver in tuina-massage is used to treat an excess pattern of the lower-energizer.

泻肺平喘[xiè fèi píng chuǎn] purging lung-fire to relieve panting ~ 法, 治疗痰热阻肺, 气道不利之喘证。 Purging lung-fire to relieve panting is employed to treat the problem caused by obstruction of the air passage by phlegm-heat.

泻剂[xiè jì] purgative formula 苦寒 ~ purgatives bitter in flavor and cold in property

泻水逐饮[xiè shuǐ zhú yǐn] removing retained water and morbid fluid

泻心[xiè xīn] purging heart-fire

泄 xiè

泄剂[xiè jì] purgative formula

泄脓血[xiè nóng xuè] passing bloody and purulent feces 痢疾可见腹痛 ~ 。 Dysentery manifests itself as an abdominal pain with passing bloody and purulent feces.

泄泻[xiè xiè] diarrhea

心辛新欣囟 XIN

心 xīn

心[xīn] heart ~ 者, 五脏六腑之主也。 The heart is the master of the zang-fu organs.

心安[xīn ān] peaceful mind ~ 理得 having an easy conscience/ ~ 即福。 A peaceful mind means blessing.

心安而不惧[xīn ān ér bù jù] not terrified and at ease when one has a peaceful mind

心包 [xīn bāo] pericardium ~ 经 Pericardium Meridian

心病还须心药医 [xīn bìng hái xū xīn yào yī] Worry is only cured by heartening news.

心病禁咸 [xīn bìng jìn xián] abstinence from salty food in patients with heart disease

心藏神 [xīn cáng shén] spirit housed in the heart

心定 [xīn dìng] mental harmony; spirit calmness ~ 则神凝 spirit calmness with attention focused

心烦 [xīn fán] vexation ~ 易怒 feeling upset and easy to flare up/ ~ 失眠为虚火内扰神明所致。Vexation and insomnia are due to the mind disturbed by fire in a deficiency condition.

心扉 [xīn fēi] heart of hearts 打开 ~ opening one's heart

心肺气虚 [xīn fèi qì xū] qi deficiency of the heart and lung

心火亢盛 [xīn huǒ kàng shèng] hyperactivity of heart-fire

心经 [xīn jīng] Heart Meridian

心静 [xīn jìng] mental tranquilization ~ 体松 mental tranquilization and body relaxation/ ~ 自然凉。So long as one keeps calm, one doesn't feel so hot.

心肝血虚 [xīn gān xuè xū] blood deficiency of the heart and liver

心合小肠 [xīn hé xiǎo cháng] heart and small intestine in pair ~ , 肺合大肠。The heart and small intestine are in pair while the lung is in pair with the large intestine.

心悸 [xīn jì] palpitation

心开窍于舌 [xīn kāi qiào yú shé] tongue, the window of the heart

心宽 [xīn kuān] carefree; open-minded ~ 体胖 carefree and contented

心劳 [xīn láo] racking one's brains ~ 勿过 not racking one's brains too much

心理健康 [xīn lǐ jiàn kāng] mental health

心脉闭阻 [xīn mài bì zǔ] obstruction of the Heart Meridian

心脾两虚 [xīn pí liǎng xū] deficiency in the heart and spleen

心气 [xīn qì] heart-qi; intention; mood; breadth of mind; ambition ~ 不顺 in a bad mood/ ~ 高 having lofty aspiration/ ~ 相随 of the same mind/ ~ 盛 exuberance of heart-qi/ ~ 虚 deficiency of heart-qi/ ~ 窄 narrow minded/ ~ 不宁则见心悸。Palpitation is seen in unsteadiness of heart-qi. / ~ 充足, 神有所归, 意念集中。Abundant heart-qi may lead to relaxing spirit and focusing mind.

心情 [xīn qíng] mood, frame of mind ~ 不佳 in a bad mood/ ~ 沉重 having a heavy heart/ ~ 复杂 having mixed feeling/ ~ 舒畅 enjoying ease of mind

心神 [xīn shén] effort; frame of mind ~ 安定 peace of mind/ ~ 不安 feeling unsettled/ ~烦乱 being irritable/ ~极耗 being very taxing on one's mind/ ~稳定 calmness/气功可调治 ~。 *Qigong* works to calm down.

心肾不交[xīn shèn bù jiāo] failure of the normal physiological coordination between heart-yang and kidney-yin 失眠主要由 ~引起的。 Failure of the normal physiological coordination between heart-yang and kidney-yin is the chief cause of insomnia.

心肾阳虚[xīn shèn yáng xū] deficiency of heart-yang and kidney-yang

心痛引背[xīn tòng yǐn bèi] heartache with the back involved

心下[xīn xià] gastric region

心下急[xīn xià jí] distress below the heart

心下痞[xīn xià pǐ] gastric fullness and hardness

心胸豁达[xīn xiōng huò dá] broad-minded ~, 不至损伤肝气。 When one is broad-minded, liver-qi will not be impaired.

心阳虚脱[xīn yáng xū tuō] collapse of heart-yang

心宜常静[xīn yí cháng jìng] calming down often 身宜常动, ~。 Do exercise frequently and calm down often.

心斋[xīn zhāi] purifying the heart; heart fast 庄子主张"坐忘""~"。 Zhuang Zi, an ancient philosopher, proposed "seating forgetting" and "purifying the heart".

心正[xīn zhèng] uprightness ~不怕邪。 If one's behavior and attitude are very moral and honest, he does not fear evils.

心主汗[xīn zhǔ hàn] sweat governed by the heart

心主神明[xīn zhǔ shén míng] heart dominating mental activities

心主血脉[xīn zhǔ xuè mài] blood and vessels governed by the heart

辛 xīn

辛[xīn] pungent, acrid 夏省苦增 ~, 以养肺气。 Eat less food bitter in taste and more food pungent in flavor to nourish lung-qi in summer.

辛甘化阳[xīn gān huà yáng] yang transformed from herbal medicinals pungent and sweet in flavor

辛开苦降[xīn kāi kǔ jiàng] herbal medicinals pungent in flavor for dispersing and those bitter in flavor for descending

辛凉解表[xīn liáng jiě biǎo] releasing an exterior pattern with herbal medicinals pungent in flavor and cool in property

辛凉平剂[xīn liáng píng jì] a moderate formula with herbal medicinals pungent in flavor and cool in property 银翘散为 ~。 The *Yinqiao* Powder is a moderate formula with medicinals pungent in flavor and cool in property.

辛凉透疹[xīn liáng tòu zhěn] inducing

eruptions with herbal medicinals pungent in flavor and cool in property 麻疹初起, 发热恶寒, 宜 ~ 。 At the initial stage of measles there presents fever and it is advisable to induce eruptions with medicinals pungent in flavor and cool in property.

辛温解表 [xīn wēn jiě biǎo] releasing an exterior pattern with herbal medicinals pungent in flavor and warm in property ~ 剂用于外感风寒表证。 Herbal medicinals pungent in flavor and warm in property are prescribed for an exterior pattern due to contraction of external wind-cold.

新 xīn

新病 [xīn bìng] recent illness

新感 [xīn gǎn] recently contracted disease

欣 xīn

欣赏 [xīn shǎng] appreciation 自我 ~ self-appreciation

欣慰 [xīn wèi] gratified 感到 ~ feeling gratified

囟 xìn

囟门 [xìn mén] fontanel ~ 闭合 closure of the fontanel/ ~ 不闭 metopism

囟填 [xìn tián] bulge of the fontanel

囟陷 [xìn xiàn] depressed fontanel

行形醒性 XING

行 xíng

行房 [xíng fáng] having sex with one's spouse ~ 过度 excessive sexual life

行气 [xíng qì] moving qi ~ 通络 moving qi to dredge meridians/ ~ 开郁 moving qi to relieve stagnancy/ ~ 宽中 moving qi to soothe the chest/ ~ 利水 moving qi for diuresis

行气活血 [xíng qì huó xuè] promoting circulation of qi and blood 两肋刺痛 可用 ~ 药。 Herbal medicinals to promote circulation of qi and blood are prescribed for hypochondrial twinge.

行气散结 [xíng qì sàn jié] moving qi to disintegrate masses ~ 可用于治疗梅核气。 Moving qi to disintegrate masses is used in treatment for globus hystericus.

行气止痛 [xíng qì zhǐ tòng] moving qi to kill pain 气滞引起的胀痛可用 ~ 药。 Distending pain due to qi stagnancy is treated with medicinals that promote qi circulation to kill pain.

行医 [xíng yī] practising medicine 世代 ~ practising medicine for generations

行坐端正 [xíng zuò duān zhèng] walking and sitting straightly

形 xíng

形不足者, 温之以气 [xíng bù zú zhě, wēn zhī yǐ qì] People with a flabby appearance should be treated with medicinals warm in nature to reinforce qi.

形苦志苦 [xíng kǔ zhì kǔ] a person who is physically tired and depressed

形苦志乐 [xíng kǔ zhì lè] a person who

is physically tired but happy

形劳而不倦[xíng láo ér bù juàn] hard manual labor yet without physical exhaustion

形乐志苦[xíng lè zhì kǔ] a person who is physically good but depressed

形乐志乐[xíng lè zhì lè] a person who is physically good and happy

形气[xíng qì] physique and qi ~ 相得 equilibrium between the physique and qi / ~ 相失 imbalance between the physique and qi

形气不足[xíng qì bù zú] poor physique

形气充[xíng qì chōng] strong physique

形气未充[xíng qì wèi chōng] undeveloped physique and qi 小儿脏腑娇嫩，~。 Infants' internal organs are always delicate because their body build and qi are not fully developed.

形神合一[xíng shén hé yī] unity of the physique and mental state; integration of body and spirit 只有达到 ~ 的境界, 才能称之为身心健康。 Only by reaching the unity of the physique and mental state can one be physically and mentally healthy.

形神共养[xíng shén gòng yǎng] building up physique and cultivating spirit

形食味[xíng sì wèi] Physique builds up with flavor (food). 精食气，~。 Essence production depends on qi transformation and physique builds up by flavor (food).

形体[xíng tǐ] figure ~ 美 physical beauty

醒 xǐng

醒脑[xǐng nǎo] resuscitation

醒脾开胃[xǐng pí kāi wèi] activating the spleen and whetting appetite

性 xìng

性高潮[xìng gāo cháo] orgasm

性格[xìng gé] nature, character, disposition 不同~ different characters / ~ 温和 having a gentle disposition

性寒[xìng hán] cold in property 石膏 ~ Gypsum is cold in property.

性冷淡[xìng lěng dàn] frigidity

性命双修[xìng mìng shuāng xiū] dual cultivation ~ 是内丹术的核心。 Dual cultivation is the core of the *Neidan* training.

性平[xìng píng] mild-natured ~ 的药 mild-natured medicinals

性热[xìng rè] hot in property ~ 之品, 善于温通经脉。 Herbal medicinals hot in property tend to warm the meridians and remove obstruction. / ~ 之药, 易伤人正气。 Hot-property medicaments easily impair healthy qi.

性生活[xìng shēng huó] sexual life

性微凉[xìng wēi liáng] slightly cool in property 菊花 ~。 Chrysanthemum is slightly cool in property.

性微温[xìng wēi wēn] slightly warm in property

性味[xìng wèi] property and flavor, nature and taste

性欲[xìng yù] libido 肾阳不足可致 ~

减退。Loss of libido is caused by deficiency of kidney-yang. /抑郁症常见~冷淡。Poor libido is often seen in patients with depression.

胸 XIONG

胸 xiōng

胸痹[xiōng bì]qi blockage in the chest

胸痞[xiōng pǐ] fullness in the chest

胸前抱球[xiōng qián bào qiú] raising two hands close to the chest as if holding a ball 站桩时，双脚与肩同宽，双手提至~。In stance training one has to stand shoulder-width apart, and raise two hands close to the chest as if holding a ball.

胸胁苦满[xiōng xié kǔ mǎn]fullness and discomfort in the chest and hypochondrium

胸宜常护[xiōng yí cháng hù] caring the chest often

胸宜常扩[xiōng yí cháng kuò] expanding one's chest often ~, 使气机通畅。Expand one's chest often to ensure good qi activity.

胸中气满[xiōng zhōng qì mǎn] suffocating

修休羞秀臭绣嗅 XIU

修 xiū

修德怡神[xiū dé yí shén] cultivating morality to gladden the heart

修炼[xiū liàn] practicing asceticism

修身养性[xiū shēn yǎng xìng] cultivating one's moral character and behaving ethically

修养[xiū yǎng] accomplishment; self-cultivation 没有~ ill cultivated/有~ well cultivated/艺术~ artistic culture

修指甲[xiū zhǐ jia]manicure

休 xiū

休克[xiū kè]shock 外伤性~ traumatic shock

休息痢[xiū xī lì]recurrent dysentery

羞 xiū

羞明[xiū míng] photophobia ~隐涩 photophobia and eye discomfort

秀 xiù

秀气[xiù qì] delicate; refined

秀色[xiù sè] beautiful scenery ~可餐 being a feast to the eye

臭 xiù

臭恶不食[xiù è bù shí] not eating smelly food

绣 xiù

绣球风[xiù qiú fēng]scrotal eczema

嗅 xiù

嗅气味[xiù qì wèi]smelling the odor of a patient, his secretion, excretion and ward

虚续蓄 XU

虚 xū

虚[xū] deficiency ~证 deficiency pattern

虚步[xū bù] flexed foot position ~推

X

掌。Push hands in a flexed foot position.

虚烦不眠[xū fán bù mián]insomnia due to vexation in a deficiency condition

虚风内动[xū fēng nèi dòng]stirring of internal wind in a deficiency condition

虚寒带下[xū hán dài xià]morbid leukorrhea due to cold in a deficiency condition

虚火[xū huǒ]fire in a deficiency condition ~上炎 flaring of fire in a deficiency condition

虚家[xū jiā]debilitated person ~忌大汗。For debilitated people it is forbidden to induce profuse sweating.

虚静恬淡[xū jìng tián dàn]peaceful and indifferent to fame and gain

虚劳[xū láo]consumptive disease ~腰痛 lower back pain in a consumptive disease/~盗汗 night sweat in a consumptive disease/~咳嗽 coughing in a consumptive disease

虚里[xū lǐ]area of the apex beat ~候宗气的盛衰。Palpation of the area of the apex beat detects increase or decrease of pectoral qi.

虚脉[xū mài]feeble pulse ~主气虚、血虚、伤津等证。Feeble pulse suggests deficiency of qi, blood and impairment of body fluids.

虚胖[xū pàng]puffiness in a deficiency condition

虚热[xū rè]fever in a deficiency condition

虚弱[xū ruò]weakness 正气不足则现~之象。Insufficiency of healthy qi manifests itself as weakness.

虚实[xū shí]deficiency and excess ~并重 laying equal stress on both the deficiency and excess conditions/真假~ true and false deficiency and excess patterns

虚实夹杂[xū shí jiā zá]simultaneous occurrence of the deficiency and excess patterns

虚损劳乏[xū sǔn láo fá]weariness due to consumption

虚邪[xū xié]pathogenic factors in a deficiency condition ~贼风，避之有时。Timely avoid the attack by pathogenic factors that take advantages of declined healthy qi.

虚阳外越[xū yáng wài yuè]outward going of yang in a deficiency condition ~可见两颧发红。Outward going of yang in a deficiency condition is marked by flushed cheeks.

虚则补其母[xū zé bǔ qí mǔ]reinforcing the mother-organ in a deficiency condition

虚则补之[xū zé bǔ zhī]reinforcing in a deficiency condition ~，实则泻之 reinforcing in a deficiency condition and reducing in an excess condition

虚胀[xū zhàng]flatulence in a deficiency condition

虚肿[xū zhǒng]edema in a deficiency condition

虚坐努责［xū zuò nǔ zé］tenesmus 气虚则可见 ~。Qi deficiency may lead to tenesmus.

续 xù

续筋接骨［xù jīn jiē gǔ］union of fracture

蓄 xù

蓄水［xù shuǐ］water accumulation

蓄血［xù xuè］blood accumulation

宣玄悬旋 XUAN

宣 xuān

宣发［xuān fā］ventilating ~ 肺气 ventilating lung-qi

宣肺平喘［xuān fèi píng chuǎn］ventilating lung-qi to relieve panting

宣剂［xuān jì］stasis or phlegm dispersing formula

宣散风热［xuān sàn fēng rè］diffusing wind-heat

宣通水道［xuān tōng shuǐ dào］dredging water passage

玄 xuán

玄府［xuán fǔ］sweat pore

悬 xuán

悬灸［xuán jiǔ］suspended moxibustion 雀啄灸为 ~ 的一种。Bird-pecking moxibustion is a kind of suspended moxibustion.

悬饮［xuán yǐn］pleural fluid retention

悬雍垂［xuán yōng chuí］uvula

旋 xuán

旋腰转脊［xuán yāo zhuǎn jǐ］moving the lower back and spine column left and right

穴血 XUE

穴 xué

穴位［xué wèi］acupoint, point ~ 埋线 acupoint thread imbedding/ ~ 注射 acupoint injection

血 xuè

血崩［xuè bēng］metrorrhagia ~ 昏暗 going off in faint with metrorrhagia

血分实热［xuè fèn shí rè］excessive heat in the blood level

血分虚热［xuè fèn xū rè］heat in the blood level in a deficiency condition

血分证［xuè fèn zhèng］pattern of the blood level, blood level disorder

血海［xuè hǎi］blood reservoir（sea）

血汗同源［xuè hàn tóng yuán］blood and sweat being of the same source 夺血者无汗，因为 ~。Diaphoresis cannot be adopted for patients who are predisposed to bleeding because blood and sweat are of the same source.

血枯［xuè kū］blood depletion

血亏经闭［xuè kuī jīng bì］amenorrhea due to blood deficiency

血离经脉［xuè lí jīng mài］escape of blood from vessels

血淋［xuè lìn］stranguria with hematuria

血能载气［xuè néng zài qì］blood carrying qi

血尿［xuè niào］hematuria

X

血气［xuè qì］blood and qi ~经络胜形则寿。One whose skin and muscles are symmetrical and coordinated enjoys longevity.

血室［xuè shì］blood chamber; uterus 热入 ~ pathogenic heat invading the uterus

血丝［xuè sī］blood streak ~痰 sputum with blood streak

血随气陷［xuè suí qì xiàn］bleeding due to sinking of qi

血脱［xuè tuō］blood exhaustion

血虚生风［xuè xū shēng fēng］wind stirred from deficiency of blood

血虚质［xuè xū zhì］type of blood-deficiency constitution ~需健脾养肝,益气生血。For people with blood-deficiency constitution it is advisable to invigorate the spleen and liver, replenish qi and generate blood.

血瘀水停［xuè yū shuǐ tíng］blood stagnation and water retention

血瘀质［xuè yū zhì］type of blood-stagnation constitution ~ 需疏肝理气,活血化瘀。For people with blood-stagnation constitution it is advisable to regulatge liver-qi, promote blood circulation to remove blood stagnation.

血痣［xuè zhì］vascular nevus

血滞［xuè zhì］impeded blood flow ~腹痛 abdominal pain due to impeded flow of blood

血肿［xuè zhǒng］hematoma

熏循汛 XUN

熏 xūn

熏法［xūn fǎ］fumigation 药物 ~ fumigation with medicinals

熏肉［xūn ròu］smoked meat, bacon

熏衣［xūn yī］fumigating clothes 沐浴 ~ fumigating clothes and taking a bath

熏蒸疗法［xūn zhēng liáo fǎ］fuming and steaming therapy

循 xún

循法［xún fǎ］touching along a meridian ~ 可促使得气。Touching along meridians may promote the arrival of qi.

循经传［xún jīng chuán］sequential meridian transmission ~ 为疾病的正常传变。Sequential meridian transmission is a normal progression of a disease.

循经取穴［xún jīng qǔ xué］acupoint selected along its own meridian

循理乐俗［xún lǐ lè sú］having conscience, kind heart and following law, and living a life according to custom

循循善诱［xún xún shàn yòu］giving guidance in a skillful and systematical fashion

循衣摸床［xún yī mō chuáng］floccillation 精亏神衰可见 ~。Floccillation is seen in a delirious patient.

汛 xùn

汛期［xùn qī］menstruation ~不宜饮

冷、提重物和剧烈运动。During menstruation it is advisable not to eat | cold foods, carry heavy load and do strenuous exercise.

Y

压押牙哑雅亚 YA

压 yā

压垫［yā diàn］pressure pad ~ 可防止骨折再移位。Using a pressure pad prevents redisplacement of a fracture.

压痛点［yā tòng diǎn］*Ashi* acupoint; tender spot

押 yā

押切法［yā qiē fǎ］nail-pressure ~ 可用于诊断和治疗疾病。The nail-pressure method can be employed in diagnosis and treatment for diseases.

押手［yā shǒu］pressing hand ~ 有固定穴位、减轻针刺疼痛和防止针身弯曲的作用。With hand pressing an acupoint is fixed, pain due to needling is relieved, and the body of a needle avoids bending.

牙 yá

牙疳［yá gān］ulcerative gingivitis

牙线［yá xiàn］dental floss ~ 不宜重复使用。Do not repeatedly use the same dental floss.

牙龈出血［yá yín chū xiě］gingival bleeding

牙龈肿痛［yá yín zhǒng tòng］swollen painful gum

哑 yǎ

哑风［yǎ fēng］apoplectic aphasia

哑嗽［yǎ sòu］cough with hoarseness

雅 yǎ

雅俗共赏［yǎ sú gòng shǎng］suiting both refined and popular tastes, appealing to all 杂技表演 ~。The acrobatic show appealed to tastes of both the refined and popular.

亚 yà

亚健康［yà jiàn kāng］sub-health 处于 ~ 状态 in a state of sub-health

咽阉言岩盐颜眼偃验厌燕 YAN

咽 yān

咽［yān］pharynx ~ 底 posterior pharyngeal wall

咽喉不利［yān hóu bù lì］discomfort of the throat

咽津［yān jīn］saliva swallowing

咽痛［yān tòng］sore throat

咽痒［yān yǎng］itchy throat

阉 yān

阉割［yān gē］castration

Y

言 yán

言语謇涩[yán yǔ jiǎn sè] dysphasia

岩 yán

岩[yán] cancer, carcinoma

盐 yán

盐炙法[yán zhì fǎ] processed with salt

颜 yán

颜[yán] face

颜面浮肿[yán miàn fú zhǒng] puffy face

眼 yǎn

眼干涩[yǎn gān sè] dry eye 多眨眼防~。Blink your eyes often to prevent dry eyes.

眼花[yǎn huā] dim eyesight

眼睑[yǎn jiǎn] eyelid ~浮肿 swollen eyelid

眼痉挛[yǎn jìng luán] ophthalmospasm ~可从肝论治。Try to treat the liver to deal with ophthalmospasm.

眼科[yǎn kē] ophthalmology

眼球[yǎn qiú] eyeball ~转动~ rotating eyeballs

眼圈[yǎn quān] eye socket 他累得~发黑。His eyes were ringed with fatigue.

眼跳[yǎn tiào] twitching of the eyelid

偃 yǎn

偃刀脉[yǎn dāo mài] knife-edge pulse

验 yàn

验方[yàn fāng] proved recipe

厌 yàn

厌食[yàn shí] having poor appetite

燕 yàn

燕（闲）居[yàn（xián）jū] leisurely living

扬疡羊阳烊仰养 YANG

扬 yáng

扬刺[yáng cì] central-square needling ~用于范围较大,病位较浅的寒痹。The central-square needling is indicated for arthralgia due to cold affecting a larger area in a mild case.

疡 yáng

疡医[yáng yī] sore and wound practitioner

羊 yáng

羊水[yáng shuǐ] amniotic fluid ~过多 excessive amniotic fluid

羊痫风[yáng xián fēng] epilepsy

阳 yáng

阳[yáng] yang ~病 disease of yang nature/ ~乘阴 yang over-acting yin

阳闭[yáng bì] coma with heat manifestations

阳病治阴[yáng bìng zhì yīn] treating the yin aspect for disease of the yang nature

阳常有余,阴常不足[yáng cháng yǒu yú, yīn cháng bù zú] yang usually being surplus while yin scanty

阳春面[yáng chūn miàn] noodles in plain sauce

阳道实[yáng dào shí] yang often in excess ~,阴道虚。Yang is often in excess while yin in deficiency.

阳刚［yáng gāng］manly 有～之气的男人 a manly man

阳光充足［yáng guāng chōng zú］adequate sunshine

阳化气［yáng huà qì］yang transforming into qi ～，阴成形。Yang transforms into qi while yin constitutes the physique.

阳黄［yáng huáng］yang jaundice ～多呈急性。Yang jaundice is an acute condition.

阳极反阴［yáng jí fǎn yīn］yin arising when yang is in extreme

阳结［yáng jié］yang constipation

阳经［yáng jīng］yang meridian

阳绝［yáng jué］yang exhaustion

阳厥［yáng jué］cold limbs or syncope due to intense heat

阳离子［yáng lí zǐ］positive ion, kation

阳面［yáng miàn］sunny side 我的卧室在～。My bedroom is on the sunny side.

阳明腑证［yáng míng fǔ zhèng］*Yangming fu*-organ excess pattern ～承气汤主之。The *Chengqi* Decoction is indicated for the *Yangming fu*-organ excess pattern.

阳明经证［yáng míng jīng zhèng］*Yangming* Meridian pattern

阳气［yáng qì］yang-qi ～盛 abundant yang-qi/～不足，寒从内生。Cold produced in the interior is due to deficiency of yang-qi. /～不足，四肢厥冷，脉微欲绝 Insufficient yang-qi leads to cold limbs and fainting pulse. /日中而～隆。At noon time yang-qi is abundant. /日西而～已虚。In the evening at sunset yang-qi is declining.

阳强［yáng qiáng］long-time erection ～滑精 long-time erection and spermatorrhea

阳跷脉［yáng qiāo mài］Yang Heel Vessel ～为连络阴经与阳经的经脉。The Yang Heel Vessel is one that links the yin and yang meridians.

阳人［yáng rén］yang-featured person

阳杀阴藏［yáng shā yīn cáng］yin concealed when yang is restrained

阳生于阴［yáng shēng yú yīn］existence of yang with yin as its prerequisite

阳胜则热［yáng shèng zé rè］excessive yang giving rise to heat manifestations

阳胜则阴病［yáng shèng zé yīn bìng］yang in excess making yin suffer

阳事［yáng shì］male sexuality

阳寿［yáng shòu］life span

阳损及阴［yáng sǔn jí yīn］impairment of yang with yin involved

阳维脉［yáng wéi mài］Yang Link Vessel ～维系人体一身之阳气。The Yang Link Vessel connects with yang-qi of the whole body.

阳痿［yáng wěi］impotence 湿热型～ impotence due to dampness-heat

阳性［yáng xìng］positive 核酸～ nucleic acid positive

阳虚水泛［yáng xū shuǐ fàn］edema due

Y

to yang deficiency

阳虚则阴盛［yáng xū zé yīn shèng］
yang deficiency leading to excessive yin

阳虚质［yáng xū zhì］type of yang-deficiency constitution ~ 需温补脾肾。For people with the type of yang-deficiency constitution it is advisable to reinforce the spleen and kidney with medicinals warm in nature.

阳在外,阴之使也［yáng zài wài , yīn zhī shǐ yě］Yang stays outside to protect yin.

阳脏［yáng zàng］zang-organs of the yang nature 心为 ~。The heart is a yang-natured zang-organ.

阳宅［yáng zhái］residence

阳中有阳［yáng zhōng yǒu yáng］yang within yang

烊 yáng

烊化［yáng huà］melting 阿胶、鹿角胶多 ~。The donkey-hide gelatin and antler glue are usually melted.

仰 yǎng

仰卧［yǎng wò］lying on one's back ~ 起坐 sit-ups

养 yǎng

养德［yǎng dé］cultivating morality 立志 ~ setting one's mind on cultivating morality/养心贵在 ~。Priority must be on cultivating virtue when one wants to be a kind person. /以 ~ 致长生。People with high moral character enjoy long life.

养耳之道［yǎng ěr zhī dào］way to keep healthy ears

养肝明目［yǎng gān míng mù］nourishing the liver to improve eyesight ~之法治疗肝血不足,血不荣目,视物不清之症. Nourishing the liver to improve eyesight is for blurred vision due to deficiency of liver-blood, which fails to nourish eyes.

养骨［yǎng gǔ］toning up bones 补骨填精髓以 ~ 强身。Health promotion and wellness is achieved by reinforcing the kidney, and replenishing essence to tone up bones.

养护阳气［yǎng hù yáng qì］protecting yang-qi

养精［yǎng jīng］enriching essence 节欲以 ~ controling one's desire for sex to enrich essence

养老［yǎng lǎo］providing for the aged ~送终。Look after one's parents in their old age and give them a proper burial after their death. /攒钱 ~ saving money for one's old age

养目之道［yǎng mù zhī dào］way to keep healthy eyes

养内［yǎng nèi］nourishing internal organs

养鸟消遣法［yǎng niǎo xiāo qiǎn fǎ］killing time by keeping pet birds

养气［yǎng qì］reinforcing qi ~ 活血 reinforcing qi and activating blood flow/ ~ 保精 reinforcing qi to preserve essence

养人［yǎng rén］being nutritious 这东西很 ~。This is very nutritious.

养神［yǎng shén］rest to attain mental tranquility 闭目 ~ sitting and relaxing with one's eyes closed/清静 ~ cultivating spirit tranquilly/修性 ~ cultivating the temperament and reposing/动以养形、静以 ~。Exercise improves physical health while rest attains mental tranquility.

养慎［yǎng shèn］cultivating healthy qi and warding off external pathogens 人能 ~，不令邪风干忤经络。One should cultivate healthy qi and resist invasion of the meridians by pathogenic wind and cold.

养生［yǎng shēng］health preservation, health promotion and wellness, life nurturing/ ~ 当以食补,治病当以药攻。Health preservation should depend on food intake while treatment for diseases should depend on medicines. / ~ 的原则和方法 principle and method of health preservation/ ~ 功 health building up qigong/ ~ 文化 wellness culture/ ~ 之道 way of life nurturing"/运动 ~ building up one's health with exercise/ ~ 有常 leading a regular life/ ~ 必须持之以恒。Health preservation requires unremitting effort. /故智者之 ~ 也,必顺四时而适寒暑。A wise man who understands health preservation can adapt himself to the temperature change in the four seasons.

养生十六宜［yǎng shēng shí liù yí］sixteen suggestions for health preservation

养胎［yǎng tāi］nourishing the fetus ~ 安胎 nourishing the fetus and preventing miscarriage/ ~ 优生 nourishing the fetus to ensure aristogenesis

养体之道［yǎng tǐ zhī dào］way to keep healthy

养胃［yǎng wèi］taking care of one's stomach

养心［yǎng xīn］protecting the heart ~ 安神 protecting the heart and calming the mind/ ~ 敛思 protecting the heart and getting rid of distracting thoughts

养性［yǎng xìng］disciplining one's temperament 存心 ~ harboring intentions and discipling the temperament

养血［yǎng xuè］enriching blood ~ 润燥 enriching blood and removing dryness/ ~ 息风 enriching blood to subside wind

养颜［yǎng yán］taking care of one's complexion

养阴［yǎng yīn］replenishing yin ~ 补血 replenishing yin and blood/ ~ 解表 replenishing yin and release an exterior pattern/ ~ 清肺 replenishing yin to clear lung-heat

腰摇药 YAO
腰 yāo

腰肌劳损［yāo jī láo sǔn］strain of

lumbar muscles 长时间弯腰可致 ~。Long-time bending causes lumbar muscle strain.

腰间盘突出 [yāo jiān pán tū chū] prolapse of the lumbar intervertebral disc 牵引复位法治疗 ~。Traction for restoration is used for prolapse of the lumbar intervertebral disc.

腰膝酸软 [yāo xī suān ruǎn] aching pain and weakness of the lower back and knees ~，不能持重 inability of carrying a heavy load because of aching pain and weakness of the lower back and knees/肾虚 ~ aching pain and weakness of the lower back and knees due to deficiency in the kidney

腰椎 [yāo zhuī] lumbar vertebra ~ 滑脱 lumbar spondylolisthesis

摇 yáo

摇法 [yáo fǎ] revolving ~ 的动作要缓和，用力要稳。The revolving maneuver is done gently with a steady force.

药 yào

药补 [yào bǔ] building up one's health by taking tonics ~ 不如食补。Diet helps more than tonics.

药材 [yào cái] medicinal substance 地道 ~ authenic medicinal substances 天然 ~ natural medicinal substances

药茶 [yào chá] medicated tea 许多人通过喝 ~ 调理身体。People like to nurse themselves by drinking medicated tea.

药方 [yào fāng] prescription

药粉 [yào fěn] medicinal powder

药膏 [yào gāo] medicinal paste; ointment

药罐法 [yào guàn fǎ] medicated cupping

药罐子 [yào guàn zi] pot for decocting herbal medicinals

药酒 [yào jiǔ] medicated wine 跌打损伤 ~ medicated wine for traumatic injury/ ~ 外擦 medicated wine for external application

药力 [yào lì] potency of medicinals 使 ~ 直达病所 guiding the potency of medicinals directly to the diseased site

药露 [yào lù] distilled medicinal liquid

药面 [yào miàn] medicinal powder

药捻子 [yào niǎn zi] medicated thread

药膳 [yào shàn] medicinal cuisine, medicated food, herbal cuisine 健脾祛湿 ~ 或可缓解肥胖病。Medicinal cuisine that reinforces the spleen and eliminates dampness may relieve obesity.

药食同源 [yào shí tóng yuán] herbal medicinal and food being of the same source 制作药膳应选取 ~ 的食材。When we want to prepare medicinal cuisine, we have to use the materials of the same source.

药苔 [yào tāi] tongue coating dyed by medicinals

药调灸 [yào tiáo jiǔ] medicinal moxibustion

药丸 [yào wán] pill; bolus

药味［yào wèi］medicinal ingredient in a formula; flavor of medicinal substance

药线［yào xiàn］medicated thread ~ 引流 drainage with medicated thread

药性［yào xìng］potency of medicinal substances ~ 强烈 strong potency of a medicinal substance/ ~ 平和 mild potency of a medicinal substance

药引［yào yǐn］extra conductive ingredient ~ 可引药直达病所。An extra conductive ingredient can guide the potency of herbal medicinals directly to the diseased site.

药用炭［yào yòng tàn］medicinal charcoal

药浴［yào yù］medicated bath ~ 方 medicated bath prescription/ ~ 是中医外治法之一。Medicated bath is one of the TCM external therapies.

药渣滓［yào zhā zǐ］dregs of a herbal decoction ~ 可以用来泡脚。The dregs of a herbal decoction can be used for soaking foot.

药枕［yào zhěn］medicated pillow

药汁炙［yào zhī zhì］processed with herbal decoction

药粥［yào zhōu］medicated congee 养生 ~ 各有特色。Each medicated congee has its own characteristics. / ~ 能益人，老年尤宜。Medicated congee is good for health, especially for the aged.

夜腋液 YE

夜 yè

夜不瞑［yè bù míng］lying awake at night 昼不精，~。When one is sleepless at night he would be listless in daytime.

夜间多尿［yè jiān duō niào］polyuria at night 老年人肾虚，~。Old people usually have polyuria at night because they are suffering from deficiency in the kidney.

夜惊［yè jīng］night terror 小儿 ~ infantile night terror

夜盲［yè máng］night blindness 肝肾阴虚常出现 ~。Yin deficiency in the liver and kidney often causes night blindness/肝血不足而致 ~。Deficiency of liver-blood results in night blindness.

夜寐不安［yè mèi bù ān］restless sleep at night 心胆气虚可出现 ~。Qi deficiency in the heart and gallbladder provokes restless sleep at night.

夜热［yè rè］fever at night

夜嗽［yè sòu］night cough 肺阴虚多见 ~。Deficiency of lung-yin usually leads to night cough.

夜啼［yè tí］morbid night crying of babies ~ 呕吐 morbid night crying and vomiting of babies

夜卧不安［yè wò bù ān］restless sleep at night

夜卧早起［yè wò zǎo qǐ］going to bed later and getting up earlier (in

Y

summer）~，无厌于日。One should go to bed later and get up earlier（in summer），and not be weary of the hot days and sunshine.

腋 yè

腋臭［yè chòu］armpit odor

腋窝［yè wō］armpit

液 yè

液脱［yè tuō］exhaustion of body fluids

一医衣依移遗颐乙以艺异易疫弈益逸呓溢意噫 YI

一 yī

一次性用针［yī cì xìng yòng zhēn］disposable needle

一夫法［yī fū fǎ］palm measurement

一服药［yī fú yào］a dose of herbal medicinals 药证相符，~即愈。A dose of herbal medicinals cures an illness if it confirms to the condition.

一息［yī xī］breathing in ~ 一呼 breathing in and out

一指禅推法［yī zhǐ chán tuī fǎ］one-finger pushing

一字开［yī zì kāi］full stretch

医 yī

医案［yī àn］case record 分析 ~ analysis of case records/~ 书写 case recording/古代 ~ case records of the ancient times

医道［yī dào］physician's skill ~ 高超 physician's excellent skill/精通 ~ knowing well of physician's skill

医工［yī gōng］practitioner in ancient times

医官［yī guān］medical official in old days

医话［yī huà］medical note；medical professional essay

医经［yī jīng］medical classics

医林［yī lín］medical circle 名遐 ~ famous in medical circles

医论［yī lùn］thesis on medicine

医史［yī shǐ］medical history

医学［yī xué］medicine

衣 yī

衣不蔽体［yī bù bì tǐ］dressed in rags

依 yī

依山傍水［yī shān bàng shuǐ］situated at the foot of a hill and beside a stream 古代的寺院一般选在 ~ 的好地方。Temples in ancient times were usually situated beside a river at the foot of a mountain.

移 yí

移精变气［yí jīng biàn qì］transforming essence into qi 古之治病，惟其 ~。In ancient times proper-healing might transform essence into qi.

移情［yí qíng］changing one's affection

遗 yí

遗精［yí jīng］seminal emission 相火妄动之 ~ seminal emission due to hyperactivity of the ministerial fire/肾虚可致 ~ 阳痿。Deficiency in the kidney results in seminal emission and impotence.

遗尿［yí niào］enuresis 肾气不固可致 ~ 。 Insecurity of kidney-qi results in enuresis.

颐 yí

颐［yí］lower cheek

颐神［yí shén］carefree and happy

颐养［yí yǎng］keeping fit ~ 天年 Take good care of oneself so as to live out one's allotted lifespan.

乙 yǐ

乙癸同源［yǐ guǐ tóng yuán］liver and kidney being of the same source

以 yǐ

以表知里［yǐ biǎo zhī lǐ］internal conditions shown in external signs

以动养形［yǐ dòng yǎng xíng］building up the physique with exercise

以毒攻毒［yǐ dú gōng dú］counteracting poison with poison

以静制动［yǐ jìng zhì dòng］stopping moving by unmoving

以静制躁［yǐ jìng zhì zào］calm against restlessness

以母为基［yǐ mǔ wéi jī］taking the mother as the basis

以情胜情［yǐ qíng shèng qíng］overcoming emotional disorder with normal emotion

以痛为输［yǐ tòng wéi shū］needling the tender spot

以形补形［yǐ xíng bǔ xíng］eating domestic animals' organs to supplement human's corresponding organs

艺 yì

艺术品［yì shù pǐn］work of art

艺术体操［yì shù tǐ cāo］artistic gymnastics

异 yì

异病同食［yì bìng tóng shí］having same meal for patients with different diseases

异病同治［yì bìng tóng zhì］treating different diseases with the same method

易 yì

易感性［yì gǎn xìng］susceptibility

易筋功［yì jīn gōng］muscle bone strengthening qigong

易惊［yì jīng］proneness to fright ~ 善恐 easily to be frightened

易怒［yì nù］having a short temper

易性［yì xìng］changing the temperament 移情 ~ 疗法 changing affection and temperament therapy

疫 yì

疫［yì］epidemic disease 仲夏行秋令，则民殃于疫。 If there is autumn-like weather in midsummer, people may die from pandemic.

疫疠［yì lì］pestilence

弈 yì

弈棋［yì qí］playing chess

益 yì

益精明目［yì jīng míng mù］replenishing essence to improve vision

益气［yì qì］reinforcing qi ~ 回阳 reinforcing qi and restoring yang/ ~ 养

Y

阴 reinforcing qi and replenishing yin

益寿延年[yì shòu yán nián] prolonging life 预防疾病, ~ 。 Prevent disease to prolong life. /科学健身可 ~ 。 Scientific fitness prolongs life.

益智[yì zhì] improving intelligence

逸 yì

逸者行之[yì zhě xíng zhī] moving qi and blood ~ 多治疗过逸气血运行不畅之证。 Moving qi and blood is adopted to treat impeded qi and blood flow because of excessive idleness.

呓 yì

呓语[yì yǔ] somniloquy 神昏 ~ coma and somniloquy

溢 yì

溢泻经血[yì xiè jīng xuè] monthly periods

溢血[yì xuè] hemorrhage

溢饮[yì yǐn] subcutaneous fluid retention

意 yì

意[yì] desire; idea

意念[yì niàn] mind activities, guided imagery ~ 法 suggestive mind focusing/ ~ 疗法 mind activity therapy/ ~ 集中 focusing the mind/ ~ 移物 psychokinesis/练气功多提倡 ~ 集中。 Qigong exercises mainly advocate focusing the mind. /心气充足, 神有所归, ~ 集中。 Abundant heart-qi may lead to relaxing spirit and focusing mind.

意气功[yì qì gōng] will-control qigong

意气相随[yì qì xiāng suí] coordinating will and qi

意守[yì shǒu] mind concentration ~ 丹田 mind concentration at Dantian/打坐时应 ~ 下丹田。 Keep the mind concentrated at the lower Dantian in meditation.

意想[yì xiǎng] visualizing ~ 无云的天空 visualizing a cloudless sky

嗌 yì

嗌[yì] pharynx ~ 痹 pharyngitis/ ~ 乳 milk vomiting

因阴音吟银龈淫引饮隐瘾 YIN

因 yīn

因地而食[yīn dì ér shí] diet with regional characters

因地制宜[yīn dì zhì yí] environmental consideration in treatment for diseases

因时而食[yīn shí ér shí] eating seasonal foodstuffs 提倡 ~ , 少吃反季节食品。 Encourage to eat more seasonal foodstuffs and few out-of-season ones.

因时而异[yīn shí ér yì] variation according to the seasonal conditions

因时养生[yīn shí yǎng shēng] health preservation with consideration of the climatic and seasonal conditions

因势利导[yīn shì lì dǎo] guiding action according to circumstance

阴 yīn

阴[yīn] yin

阴闭［yīn bì］coma with cold manifestations

阴户［yīn hù］vulva

阴黄［yīn huáng］yin jaundice

阴绝［yīn jué］yin exhaustion

阴离子［yīn lí zǐ］negative ion, anion

阴平阳秘［yīn píng yáng mì］balance between yin and yang

阴器［yīn qì］genitals

阴跷脉［yīn qiāo mài］Yin Heel Vessel

阴人［yīn rén］yin-featured person

阴柔［yīn róu］graceful and restrained

阴胜则寒［yīn shèng zé hán］excessive yin giving rise to cold manifestations

阴胜则阳病［yīn shèng zé yáng bìng］yin in excess making yang suffer

阴损及阳［yīn sǔn jí yáng］impairment of yin with yang involved

阴挺［yīn tǐng］prolapse of the uterus

阴维脉［yīn wéi mài］Yin Link Vessel

阴邪［yīn xié］pathogenic factors of the yin nature

阴虚［yīn xū］yin deficiency ～盗汗 night sweating due to yin deficiency

阴虚动风［yīn xū dòng fēng］yin deficiency with stirring of wind

阴虚则阳亢［yīn xū zé yáng kàng］yin deficiency with yang hyperactivity

阴虚质［yīn xū zhì］type of yin deficiency constitution ～需养阴降火，滋补肝肾。For people with the type of yin-deficiency constitution, it is advisable to replenish yin to bring down fire and reinforce the liver and kidney.

阴阳［yīn yáng］yin and yang ～不和 disharmony between yin and yang／～互根 interdependence between yin and yang／～交 interlocking of yin and yang／～离决 divorce of yin from yang／～两虚 deficiency of both yin and yang／～配穴法 yin-yang acupoint combination／～胜复 alternation of excess and deficiency between yin and yang／～失调 imbalance between yin and yang／～消长 wax and wane of yin and yang／～协调 harmonious coexistence of yin and yang／～学说 theory of yin and yang／～易 yin-yang transmission／～鱼 yin-yang, the symbol of two fishes—one dark with a light eye and one light with a dark eye／～转化 mutual transformation between yin and yang／人由～二气交感而成。Humans come from the meeting and fusing of yin-qi and yang-qi of Heaven and Earth.／～数之可十，推之可百；数之可千，推之可万。Manifestations of yin and yang may present in ten, a hundred, a thousand or even ten thousand ways.／～者，天地之道也。yin-yang, the law of nature／～者，万物之始。yin-yang, the origin of all things／～平衡维持着正常的生命活动。Normal life activities depend on the balance between yin and yang.／～之要，阳密乃固。Strong defensive yang in the exterior ensures stable yin in the interior.

Y

阴阳闭膈[yīn yáng bì gé] separation between yin and yang.

阴阳和调之人[yīn yáng hé tiáo zhī rén] a person with balanced yin and yang

阴阳适中[yīn yáng shì zhōng] yin-yang balance

阴痒[yīn yǎng] pruritus vulvae

阴液[yīn yè] yin fluid ~ 亏损 consumption of yin fluid

阴在内,阳之守也[yīn zài nèi, yáng zhī shǒu yě] yin remaining in the interior, being the basis of yang

阴脏[yīn zàng] zang-organ of the yin nature

阴宅[yīn zhái] graveyard

阴之所生,本在五味[yīn zhī suǒ shēng, běn zài wǔ wèi] source of human yin coming from our diet and the five flavors

阴之五宫,伤在五味[yīn zhī wǔ gōng, shāng zài wǔ wèi] the five zang-organs often injured by over-eating

阴中有阴[yīn zhōng yǒu yīn] yin within yin

阴中之阳[yīn zhōng zhī yáng] yang within yin

阴肿[yīn zhǒng] swollen vulva

音 yīn

音哑[yīn yǎ] hoarseness

音乐[yīn yuè] music ~ 疗法 music therapy/~ 安神法 tranquilization with the music therapy/~ 养生 musical health preservation

吟 yín

吟诗[yín shī] reciting a poem ~ 作画 reciting poems and painting

银 yín

银针[yín zhēn] silver needle

龈 yín

龈[yín] gum

淫 yín

淫邪不能惑其心[yín xié bù néng huò qí xīn] Strong will is not disturbed by any obscene and wicked act

引 yǐn

引痘法[yǐn dòu fǎ] human variolation

引火归原[yǐn huǒ guī yuán] leading fire to its origin ~法,治疗肾火上升的方法。Leading fire to its origin is to direct ascendant kidney-fire downward.

引经报使[yǐn jīng bào shǐ] directing medicinal potency to the diseased meridian or site

引药[yǐn yào] medicinals that guide other medicinal potency to the lesion

引子[yǐn zi] medicinals that strengthen other medicinals' potency

饮 yǐn

饮[yǐn] cold herbal decoction; retained morbid fluid

饮片[yǐn piàn] processed medicinal substances, herbs prepared for ingestion

饮食[yǐn shí] food and drink ~ 定量 eating fixed quantity of food each time/～定量，饥饱适中。Eating fixed quantity of food each time, neither hungry nor too full. /～自倍，肠胃乃伤。Overeating is extremely harmful to health because it injures the stomach and intestines.

饮食不节[yǐn shí bù jié] improper diet ～,失之调养。Health is impaired by improper diet.

饮食禁忌[yǐn shí jìn jì] diet taboos 服用一些中药时可能有～。Abstain from some kinds of food when taking certain herbal medicinals.

饮食均衡[yǐn shí jūn héng] maintaining a balanced diet

饮食劳倦[yǐn shí láo juàn] improper diet and fatigue

饮食疗法[yǐn shí liáo fǎ] dietotherapy ～治百病。Dietotherapy cures illnesses.

饮食六宜[yǐn shí liù yí] six good habits at meals

饮食清淡[yǐn shí qīng dàn] light food 老年人宜～。The aged need light food.

饮食养生[yǐn shí yǎng shēng] health preservation with diet

饮食宜禁[yǐn shí yí jìn] food good or food harmful to health

饮食以时[yǐn shí yǐ shí] having meals on schedule ～,身必无灾。Having meals on schedule keeps serious illness away.

饮食有节[yǐn shí yǒu jié] proper and balanced meal

饮汤食肉[yǐn tāng shí ròu] taking both the soup and meat

饮停心包[yǐn tíng xīn bāo] morbid fluid retained in the pericardium

饮心痛[yǐn xīn tòng] stomachache due to morbid fluid retained in the stomach

饮玉泉[yǐn yù quán] swallowing saliva

饮证[yǐn zhèng] morbid fluid pattern

隐 yǐn
隐痛[yǐn tòng] dull pain

瘾 yǐn
瘾疹[yǐn zhěn] hives

婴迎营瘿硬 YING

婴 yīng
婴幼湿疹[yīng yòu shī zhěn] infantile eczema

迎 yíng
迎风[yíng fēng] against the wind ～流泪 tears running irritated by wind/～流泪多由肝肾不足或肝经郁热所致。Tears running irritated by wind is due to lowered functioning of the liver and kidney, or stagnated heat in the Liver Meridian.

迎随补泻[yíng suí bǔ xiè] directional reinforcement and reduction

营 yíng
营分[yíng fēn] nutritive level ～证 nutritive level pattern

营气[yíng qì] nutritive qi

营卫不和［yíng wèi bù hé］disharmony between the nutritive level and defensive level

营血［yíng xuè］nutritive-blood

瘿 yǐng

瘿［yǐng］goiter ~ 痈 thyroiditis

硬 yìng

硬气功［yìng qì gōng］hard *qigong*

痈涌勇用 YONG

痈 yōng

痈［yōng］abscess；carbuncle ~ 疡剂 formulas for treating abscess and ulcer

涌 yǒng

涌吐［yǒng tǔ］emetic method 酸苦 ~。 Medicinals sour and bitter in flavor induce vomiting.

勇 yǒng

勇怯人［yǒng qiè rén］a brave or timid person；a person with a strong or weak physique

勇者［yǒng zhě］bravery people；people with strong physique ~ 气行则已，怯者则着而为病也。Those with strong physique will not fall ill because qi in their body flows normally, while those with weak physique will fall ill because qi in their body becomes stagnant.

用 yòng

用寒远寒［yòng hán yuǎn hán］Avoid giving medicinals and food cold in nature in cold weather.

用热远热［yòng rè yuǎn rè］Avoid giving medicinals and food hot in nature in hot weather.

忧幽由油游疣有右幼 YOU

忧 yōu

忧［yōu］melancholy ~ 伤肺 lung impaired by melancholy/ ~ 则气郁。 Melancholy causes qi stagnation.

忧愁［yōu chóu］worried ~ 思虑即伤心。Melancholy and worry beyond measure impair the heart.

幽 yōu

幽门［yōu mén］pylorus

由 yóu

由表及里［yóu biǎo jí lǐ］knowing the interior through the external manifestations

由表入里［yóu biǎo rù lǐ］progress of a disease from the exterior to the interior

由动入静［yóu dòng rù jìng］from motion to stillness

由里出表［yóu lǐ chū biǎo］progress of a disease from the interior to the exterior

由虚转实［yóu xū zhuǎn shí］deficiency pattern developing to an excess pattern

油 yóu

油膏［yóu gāo］ointment

油汗［yóu hàn］oily sweat

游 yóu

游风［yóu fēng］hives

游走痛［yóu zǒu tòng］wandering pain

Y

疣 yóu

疣疮[yóu chuāng]verruca

疣赘[yóu zhuì]common wart 扁平 ~ flat wart

有 yǒu

有病早治[yǒu bìng zǎo zhì]timely treatment

有根[yǒu gēn]existence of kidney-qi

有汗[yǒu hàn]sweating

有神[yǒu shén]full of vitality

右 yòu

右病刺左[yòu bìng cì zuǒ] acupuncture applied to the left to treat disorders on the right

幼 yòu

幼科[yòu kē]pediatrics

瘀鱼瑜与予伛雨禹语育浴欲遇郁 YU

瘀 yū

瘀斑[yū bān]ecchymosis

瘀热[yū rè]stagnant heat

瘀伤[yū shāng] contusion with ecchymosis

瘀血[yū xuè] blood stasis ~ 郁滞 existence of blood stasis

瘀阻胞宫[yū zǔ bāo gōng]blood stagnation(stasis)in the uterus

瘀阻冲任[yū zǔ chōng rèn]blood stagnation (stasis) in the Thoroughfare Vessel and Conception Vessel

鱼 yú

鱼际[yú jì]thenar eminence

鱼翔脉[yú xiáng mài]fish-swimming pulse

鱼盐之地[yú yán zhī dì] place by the sea, a place rich in fish and salt

瑜 yú

瑜伽[yú jiā] yoga ~ 睡眠法 yoga sleep exercise/练习 ~ 可提高身体柔韧度。Yoga helps improve body's pliability.

与 yǔ

与肩同宽[yǔ jiān tóng kuān]shoulder width apart

与人为善[yǔ rén wéi shàn] aiming at helping others out of good will

予 yǔ

予而勿夺[yǔ ér wù duó] giving more and taking less 生而勿杀, ~ ,赏而勿罚,此春气之应,养生之道也。Promote growth instead of destruction, give more and take less, reward more and punish less. This is in accordance with the principle of springtime to nurture and it is the way to keep fit.

伛 yǔ

伛偻[yǔ lǚ]hunchback

雨 yǔ

雨露[yǔ lù] rain and dew; kindness

雨水[yǔ shuǐ] Rain Water ~ 之时应养护脾脏。On the day of Rain Water it is better to nurse the spleen.

雨泽丰沛[yǔ zé fēng pèi] adequate rainfall

禹 yǔ

禹步[yǔ bù] Yu's Footwork ~ 是道士

Y

在作法事时常用的一种步法动作。
The Yu's Footwork is usually adopted by Taoists when they are doing religious service.

语 yǔ

语迟[yǔ chí] baby retardation in speech

语声[yǔ shēng] voice ~低微 faint voice/ ~謇涩 slurred speech/ ~重浊 deep and harsh voice

育 yù

育阴[yù yīn] replenishing yin ~潜阳 replenishing yin and subduing yang

浴 yù

浴[yù] bath

浴鼻锻炼[yù bí duàn liàn] nose bathed with cold water ~可改善鼻黏膜的血液循环,预防感冒及呼吸道其他疾患。Nose bathed with cold water can improve blood circulation of the nasal mucosa, prevent common cold and other respiratory diseases.

浴面[yù miàn] rubbing face ~养生 rubbing face to keep healthy/ ~能够改善面部血液循环,美容养颜。Rubbing face helps promote facial blood circulation for facial beauty.

欲 yù

欲不可绝[yù bù kě jué] no asceticism ~,顺应天乐。Enjoy natural pleasure and do not practice asceticism.

欲不可强[yù bù kě qiáng] avoiding sexual overindulgence

欲不可早[yù bù kě zǎo] not having sex too early

欲不可纵[yù bù kě zòng] not indulging in sexual pleasure

欲传[yù chuán] progress of an exterior pattern

欲合先离[yù hé xiān lí] separation first, union second

欲火内动[yù huǒ nèi dòng] burning with sexual desire

欲有所忌[yù yǒu suǒ jì] taboos in sexual life

遇 yù

遇溺便溺[yù niào biàn niào] urinating upon need

郁 yù

郁火[yù huǒ] stagnant fire

郁冒[yù mào] oppressive feeling with dizziness

郁痰[yù tán] lingering phlegm ~为痰气互结,治宜理气化痰。Lingering phlegm results from union of phlegm and qi, and it is advisable to regulate qi flow and resolve phlegm in treatment.

郁证[yù zhèng] depression; stagnation pattern

渊元园原远 YUAN

渊 yuān

渊疽[yuān jū] submaxillary tuberculosis

元 yuán

元府[yuán fǔ] sweat pore

元气[yuán qì] original qi; body

resistance ~ 大伤 severe impairment of original qi/颐养 ~ taking good care of original qi

元神之府［yuán shén zhī fǔ］house of mentality

元阳［yuán yáng］kidney-yang

元阴［yuán yīn］kidney-yin 先天 ~ innate kidney-yin

园 yuán

园艺［yuán yì］horticulture ~ 养生 health preservation with horticulture

原 yuán

原络配穴［yuán luò pèi xué］combined selection of the Yuan-source acupoint and collateral acupoint

原穴［yuán xué］Yuan-source acupoint

远 yuǎn

远道取穴［yuǎn dào qǔ xué］selection of distal acupoint

远近配穴［yuǎn jìn pèi xué］selection of both distal and proximal acupoints

远眺［yuǎn tiào］looking far into the distance 登高 ~ looking far into the distance from a high place/经常 ~ 可以保护视力。Looking far into the distance helps protect vision.

远足［yuǎn zú］going on an outing 春季养生宜 ~ 。Going on an outing in spring helps keep fit.

月阅越 YUE

月 yuè

月经［yuè jīng］menstruation, periods ~ 病 menopathy/ ~ 不调 irregular menstruation/ ~ 过多 menorrhagia/ ~ 过少 oligomenorrhea/ ~ 后期 delayed menstrual cycle/ ~ 先后不定期 menstruation at irregular intervals/ ~ 先行 preceded menstrual cycle

月满无补［yuè mǎn wú bǔ］Supplementation methods should be forbidden when the moon is full.

月生无泻［yuè shēng wú xiè］Draining methods should be avoided when the moon begins to rise.

阅 yuè

阅读［yuè dú］reading 锻炼益身，~ 益思。Sports exercise is good for health, and reading improves intelligence. / ~ 使人充实。Reading makes one a full life.

越 yuè

越经传［yuè jīng chuán］skipping meridian transmission

越医学［yuè yī xué］traditional Vietnamese medicine

晕云运熨 YUN

晕 yūn

晕血［yūn xuè］blood phobia

晕针［yūn zhēn］faint during acupuncture treatment

云 yún

云雾移睛［yún wù yí jīng］hyalosis

Y

云翳[yún yì]nebula

运 yùn

运动养生[yùn dòng yǎng shēng] exercise regimen

运化[yùn huà] transportation and transformation 脾主 ~ transportation and transformation governed by the spleen

运睛[yùn jīng] moving eyeballs ~ 有闭目和开目 ~ 两种,是气功功法之一。Moving eyeballs when the eyes are open or closed is a *qigong* exercise.

运气[yùn qì] directing qi movement ~ 是气功锻炼的重要步骤。Directing qi movement is an important method in *qigong* exercise.

熨 yùn

熨法[yùn fǎ] ironing with a hot medicinal compress

熨目[yùn mù] warming the eyes

熨药[yùn yào]hot medicinal compress

Z

杂 ZA

杂 zá

杂病[zá bìng]miscellaneous disease 内伤 ~ miscellaneous diseases due to internal injury

杂医科[zá yī kē] specialty of miscellaneous medicine

杂症[zá zhèng]miscellaneous disease

再在 ZAI

再 zài

再传[zài chuán]repeated transmission

在 zài

在泉[zài quán]terrestrial effect

赞 ZAN

赞 zàn

赞刺[zàn cì] repeated shallow needling

脏藏 ZANG

脏 zàng

脏[zàng]*zang*-organ

脏毒[zàng dú] bloody feces; perianal abscess; dysentery ~ 便血 bloody feces due to heat in the stomach and intestines

脏腑[zàng fǔ] *zang-fu* organ ~ 相合 interaction among the organs/调和 ~ harmonizing the *zang* and *fu* organs, regulating the function of the *zang-fu* organs

脏腑辨证 [zàng fǔ biàn zhèng] differentiation of patterns according to the pathological changes of the *zang-fu* organs

脏会 [zàng huì] influential acupoint of the *zang*-organ

脏气 [zàng qì] qi of the *zang*-organ ~ 逆乱 disturbed qi of the *zang*-organ/ ~ 衰微 declined qi of the *zang*-organ/ ~ 衰微是病情危重之象。Declined qi of the *zang*-organ is a critical condition.

脏象 [zàng xiàng] organ manifestation ~ 思维模式 thinking model of the organ manifestations

脏躁 [zàng zào] hysteria

藏 zàng

藏密 [zàng mì] Tantric Buddhism

藏香 [zàng xiāng] Tibetan joss stick ~ 工艺 craftsmanship of the Tibetan joss stick/藏香多用于佛教的祭祀活动。The Tibetan joss sticks are often used in the Buddhist ceremony.

藏药 [zàng yào] Tibetan medicament

藏医学 [zàng yī xué] Tibetan medicine

早燥噪 ZAO

早 zǎo

早期 [zǎo qī] early stage ~ 诊断 early diagnosis ~ 症状 early symptoms

早衰 [zǎo shuāi] senilism

早衰发白 [zǎo shuāi fà bái] premature grey hair 肾精先天不足或后天消耗过度可导致 ~。Premature grey hair is caused by deficiency of inbred kidney-essence or excessive consumption of acquired kidney-essence.

早卧早起 [zǎo wò zǎo qǐ] early to bed and early rise ~，与鸡俱兴 One should rest and wake up early with the crowing roosters.

早泄 [zǎo xiè] premature ejaculation

燥 zào

燥 [zào] dry；dryness

燥火 [zào huǒ] dryness-fire ~ 阴虚 yin deficiency due to dryness-fire

燥结 [zào jié] constipation

燥咳 [zào ké] irritating dry cough

燥气 [zào qì] dryness ~ 伤肺。Dryness impairs the lung.

燥湿 [zào shī] eliminating dampness with medicinals dry in property

燥苔 [zào tāi] dry fur

燥痰 [zào tán] sticky sputum

燥邪犯肺 [zào xié fàn fèi] invasion of the lung by dryness

噪 zào

噪声污染 [zào shēng wū rǎn] noise pollution 居处宜远离 ~。Inhabited environment should be free of noise pollution.

择 ZE

择 zé

择时而食 [zé shí ér shí] having different diet in different seasons

Z

贼 ZEI
贼 zéi
贼风[zéi fēng]pathogenic wind ~伤人，多乘人之虚。Taking advantages of declined healthy qi, pathogenic wind launches an attack.

贼邪[zéi xié]pathogenic factor

增憎 ZENG
增 zēng
增液润下[zēng yè rùn xià]promoting secretion of body fluids to move bowels

增智[zēng zhì] improving intelligence
憎 zēng
憎寒[zēng hán]aversion to cold

扎乍痄 ZHA
扎 zhā
扎针[zhā zhēn] inserting a needle
乍 zhà
乍疏乍数[zhà shū zhà shuò]irregular pulse rhythm 脉搏~,见于气血即将消亡,病属垂危。Irregular pulse rhythm seen in depletion of qi and blood is a critical condition.
痄 zhà
痄腮[zhà sāi]mumps

斋 ZHAI
斋 zhāi
斋戒[zhāi jiè] fasting ~是道家的法门。Fasting is a Taoist way.

谵战站 ZHAN
谵 zhān
谵语[zhān yǔ]delirium 高热所致神昏 ~。High fever results in unconsciousness and delirium.
战 zhàn
战汗[zhàn hàn]chilly perspiration

战栗[zhàn lì]shivering with cold
站 zhàn
站桩功[zhàn zhuāng gōng] stance training qigong ~能恢复体力。The stance training qigong can recover one's strength.

掌杖胀瘴 ZHANG
掌 zhǎng
掌按法[zhǎng àn fǎ]palm pressing

掌心向下[zhǎng xīn xiàng xià]turning palms face-down
杖 zhàng
杖伤[zhàng shāng] flogging injury
胀 zhàng
胀[zhàng] distension ~满 distension and fullness ~气 flatulence ~痛 distending pain
瘴 zhàng
瘴毒[zhàng dú]miasm ~疫疠 miasm or communicable subtropical disease/山岚 ~ miasm from mountains

瘴疟[zhàng nüè]malignant malaria

瘴气[zhàng qì] miasm

Z

朝 ZHAO
朝 zhāo
朝夕［zhāo xī］all the time ~ 相处 together from morning till night

折赭 ZHE
折 zhé
折骨手法［zhé gǔ shǒu fǎ］osteoclasis

折疡［zhé yáng］fracture complicated by infection

赭 zhě
赭黑舌［zhě hēi shé］ochre ink tongue ~ 表示肾阴将绝,病危。Ochre ink tongue suggests exhaustion of kidney-yin and a critical condition.

针真诊疹枕振镇阵 ZHEN
针 zhēn
针刺［zhēn cì］acupuncture, needling ~ 角度 angle of needle insertion/ ~ 效果 acupuncture effect

针刀医学［zhēn dāo yī xué］acupotomy

针法［zhēn fǎ］acupuncture manipulation

针灸［zhēn jiǔ］acupuncture and moxibustion ~ 美容 facial beauty with acupuncture and moxibustion

针挑疗法［zhēn tiǎo liáo fǎ］needle-pricking therapy

针眼［zhēn yǎn］stye

真 zhēn
真寒假热［zhēn hán jiǎ rè］cold pattern with pseudo-heat

真火［zhēn huǒ］kidney-fire

真气［zhēn qì］original qi 恬淡虚无, ~ 从之。When one is indifferent to fame and gain and entering the state of emptiness, original qi can be replenished and preserved.

真热假寒［zhēn rè jiǎ hán］heat pattern with pseudo-cold

真实假虚证［zhēn shí jiǎ xū zhèng］excess pattern with pseudo-deficiency

真水［zhēn shuǐ］kidney-yin ~ 亏竭 extreme consumption of kidney-yin

真息［zhēn xī］gentle abdominal breathing in *qigong* exercise

真心痛［zhēn xīn tòng］angina pectoris

真虚假实证［zhēn xū jiǎ shí zhèng］deficiency pattern with pseudo-excess

真阴［zhēn yīn］kidney-yin ~ 内损失血 hemorrhage due to impairment of kidney-yin

真元下虚［zhēn yuán xià xū］insufficiency of kidney-yang

真脏脉［zhēn zàng mài］*zang*-organ exhaustion pulse ~ 外显,多表现此脏精气衰败之重症。*Zang*-organ exhaustion pulse suggests a critical condition with decaying essence of the organ itself.

诊 zhěn
诊尺肤［zhěn chǐ fū］palpation of the forearm skin

诊断［zhěn duàn］diagnosis 中医 ~ 学 traditional Chinese diagnosis

Z

诊法［zhěn fǎ］diagnostic method 中医
~包括四诊。The diagnostic method
in traditional Chinese medicine
includes four examinations.

诊籍［zhěn jí］diagnostic record

诊脉［zhěn mài］pulse-taking ~辨寒热
虚实。With pulse-taking patterns of
cold, heat, deficiency and excess can
be identified.

诊指纹［zhěn zhǐ wén］examining
superficial venules of the index
finger tip 小儿病，多~。When
infants fall ill, the superficial
venules of the index finger tip is
usually examined.

疹 zhěn

疹［zhěn］rash, eruption

枕 zhěn

枕与肩平［zhěn yǔ jiān píng］keeping a
pillow even with the shoulder ~，即仰
卧亦觉安舒。If a pillow is placed
even with the shoulder, one may
enjoy a comfortable sleep when he lies
on his back.

振 zhèn

振法［zhèn fǎ］vibrating

振寒［zhèn hán］chilly shiver

镇 zhèn

镇肝潜阳［zhèn gān qián yáng］
soothing the liver to check excessive
liver-yang ~法用于肝阳上亢之证。
Soothing the liver to check excessive
liver-yang is used to treat its
hyperactivity.

镇惊［zhèn jīng］relieving convulsion ~
安神 relieving convulsion and calming
the mind

镇痉［zhèn jìng］relieving muscular
spasm 息风 ~ subsiding internal wind
to relieve muscular spasm

镇静［zhèn jìng］tranquilizing ~安神
tranquilizing and calming the mind

镇咳［zhèn ké］relieving cough;
preventing cough ~化痰 relieving
cough and resolving phlegm

阵 zhèn

阵发痛［zhèn fā tòng］paroxysmal pain

癥怔整正证症郑 ZHENG

癥 zhēng

癥瘕［zhēng jiǎ］abdominal mass ~积
聚 abdominal masses

怔 zhēng

怔忡［zhēng chōng］severe palpitation

整 zhěng

整体观念［zhěng tǐ guān niàn］holistic
concept ~是中医特色之一。The
holistic concept is one of the
features of traditional Chinese
medicine.

正 zhèng

正当年［zhèng dāng nián］prime of
one's life

正气［zhèng qì］healthy qi, body
resistance ~存内，邪不可干。
Healthy qi keeping inside defeats any

invasion by pathogenic factors. / ~ 凛然 with awe-inspiring righteousness

正色[zhèng sè] normal complexion

正邪[zhèng xié] healthy qi and pathogenic factors ~相争 struggle between healthy qi and pathogenic factors

正性［zhèng xìng］ improving moral character; correcting one's character

正治[zhèng zhì] routine treatment

证 zhèng

证候[zhèng hòu] pattern, syndrome ~分析 pattern analysis

证型[zhèng xíng] type of pattern ~划分 classification of patterns

症 zhèng

症状[zhèng zhuàng] symptom 主要 ~ prime symptoms

郑 zhèng

郑声[zhèng shēng] unconscious fading murmuring

支脂知肢直职止指趾至志治栉致智炙制痔滞稚 ZHI

支 zhī

支膈[zhī gé] diaphragmatic stagnation

支节烦疼［zhī jié fán téng］ limb arthralgia

支饮[zhī yǐn] thoracic retained morbid fluid

支饮家［zhī yǐn jiā］ patient with thoracic retained morbid fluid

脂 zhī

脂瘤[zhī liú] lipoma

脂人[zhī rén] obese person

知 zhī

知音[zhī yīn] soul mate

知足［zhī zú］ being content with one's lot ~ 常乐。Happiness lies in contentment. / 他从不 ~。He is never content.

知足谦和［zhī zú qiān hé］ being content with one's lot and modesty ~有益于老年人身心健康。When they are content with their lot and modesty, the old people may be sound in body and mind.

肢 zhī

肢节宜常摇［zhī jié yí cháng yáo］ moving joints frequently ~ ,因为这样能保持气血运行通畅。Frequent moving joints is good for smooth flow of qi and blood.

直 zhí

直接灸[zhí jiē jiǔ] direct moxibustion

直中[zhí zhòng] direct attack

职 zhí

职场养生［zhí chǎng yǎng shēng］ health preservation in the workplace, vocational health preservation

止 zhǐ

止咳［zhǐ ké］ relieving cough ~ 平喘 relieving cough and panting

止渴[zhǐ kě] quenching thirst 清热 ~ clearing heat to quench thirst

止怒莫若诗[zhǐ nù mò ruò shī] better to recite poems to abate one's anger

Z

~ , 去忧莫若乐。It is better to recite poems to abate one's anger, or to listen to music to get rid of worries.

止痛[zhǐ tòng] relief of pain, analgesia ~ 药 analgesics

止息[zhǐ xī] pause in breathing

止血[zhǐ xuè] arrest of bleeding, hemostasis ~ 药 hemostatics

指 zhǐ

指按法[zhǐ àn fǎ] finger pressing

指纹[zhǐ wén] superficial venule of the index finger; fingerprint

趾 zhǐ

趾[zhǐ] toe

至 zhì

至道[zhì dào] best path to health preservation

志 zhì

志[zhì] will, mental power by which a person can direct his thoughts and actions ~ 同道合 sharing common ideas/ ~ 士仁人 people with high ideals/ ~ 向 aspiration

志闲而少欲[zhì xián ér shǎo yù] People with lofty aspiration have a pure heart and few worldly desires.

治 zhì

治病求本[zhì bìng qiú běn] searching for the root cause of a disease

治未病[zhì wèi bìng] prevention before disease arising, prevention first 圣人不治已病 ~ 。Sages do not seek treatment only after they fall ill, but do active prevention while being healthy. / 中医强调 ~ 。Traditional Chinese medicine has always put stress on prevention first.

治则[zhì zé] treating principle 治法 ~ treating method and principle

栉 zhì

栉发[zhì fà] combing hair

致 zhì

致虚极,守静笃[zhì xū jí, shǒu jìng dǔ] trying to be in an extreme emptiness of mind and keeping oneself in a state of stillness

智 zhì

智齿[zhì chǐ] wisdom tooth

智者乐[zhì zhě lè] wise man being happy ~ , 仁者寿。A wise man is happy, and a good man enjoys a long life.

炙 zhì

炙[zhì] frying with liquid

制 zhì

制化[zhì huà] restraint and transformation

制霜[zhì shuāng] crystallizing or powdering

制宜[zhì yí] adaptation to different situations

痔 zhì

痔疮[zhì chuāng] hemorrhoid, pile

滞 zhì

滞产[zhì chǎn] prolonged labor

滞颐[zhì yí] wet cheek

滞针［zhì zhēn］stuck needle ~ 不行。 The needle is stuck and difficult to withdraw.

稚 zhì

稚气［zhì qì］childishness 一脸 ~ an innocent-looking

稚阳稚阴［zhì yáng zhì yīn］premature yang and yin 小儿为 ~ 之体 Babies have a physique of premature yang and yin.

中忠终忪肿踵中重 ZHONG

中 zhōng

中草药［zhōng cǎo yào］Chinese herbal medicinals ~ 学 Chinese materia medica

中恶［zhōng è］attack by noxious factor

中国医药学［zhōng guó yī yào xué］ traditional Chinese medicine, ~ 是一个伟大的宝库, 应当努力发掘, 加以提高。Traditional Chinese medicine is a great treasure house, which should be explored and developed.

中焦如沤［zhōng jiāo rú òu］The middle-energizer works to macerate.

中气［zhōng qì］qi of the middle-energizer ~ 不足 insufficient qi of the middle-energizer

中西汇通派［zhōng xī huì tōng pài］ School of Integrated Traditional Chinese and Western Medicine

中消［zhōng xiāo］wasting-thirst disorder with the middle-energizer involved

中药［zhōng yào］Chinese medicinals ~ 材 Chinese medicinal substances

中医［zhōng yī］traditional Chinese medicine, Chinese medicine; practitioner of traditional Chinese medicine

中指同身寸［zhōng zhǐ tóng shēn cùn］ middle finger proportional body-cun measurement ~ 为四肢的取穴方法。 The middle finger proportional body-cun measurement is a way to select acupoints on limbs.

忠 zhōng

忠厚［zhōng hòu］sincere and kind-hearted ~ 待人 sincere and kind to people

终 zhōng

终老［zhōng lǎo］living out one's years ~ 故乡 spending remaining years in hometown

忪 zhōng

忪悸［zhōng jì］severe palpitation

肿 zhǒng

肿胀［zhǒng zhàng］swelling; general edema ~ 舌 swollen tongue

踵 zhǒng

踵息［zhǒng xī］leading qi to the sole

中 zhòng

中毒［zhòng dú］poisoning

中风［zhòng fēng］apoplexy, stroke ~ 不语 aphasia from apoplexy/ ~ 后遗症 sequelae of apoplexy/~ 昏迷 apoplectic coma/ ~ 前兆症 predrome of stroke

Z

中寒［zhòng hán］syncope due to cold

中经络［zhòng jīng luò］apoplexy with the meridian and collateral involved

中客［zhòng kè］convulsive seizure induced by terror in children

中暑［zhòng shǔ］sunstroke, heatstroke ～虚脱 collapse in sunstroke

重 zhòng

重剂［zhòng jì］heavy formula

重身［zhòng shēn］pregnancy

重听［zhòng tīng］hardness of hearing

重养脾胃［zhòng yǎng pí wèi］special attention paid to the spleen and stomach

重镇安神［zhòng zhèn ān shén］anchoring the mind with weighty medicinal substances

周肘皱昼 ZHOU

周 zhōu

周天［zhōu tiān］cosmic orbit, heavenly circuit 打通 ～ conducing qi circulation through the Conception Vessel and the Governor Vessel／大 ～ macro-cosmic orbit

肘 zhǒu

肘［zhǒu］elbow ～部伤筋 injury to the elbow soft tissues／～后 outer margin of the elbow

皱 zhòu

皱［zhòu］wrinkle ～脚 puffy feet with thickened skin

昼 zhòu

昼不精［zhòu bù jīng］listless in daytime

侏诸潴竹逐主煮助驻祝疰 ZHU

侏 zhū

侏儒［zhū rú］dwarf

诸 zhū

诸风掉眩，皆属于肝［zhū fēng diào xuàn, jiē shǔ yú gān］Dizziness and shaking of the head and limbs are caused by stirring of liver-wind.

诸寒之而热者取之阴［zhū hán zhī ér rè zhě qǔ zhī yīn］Replenishing kidney-yin is adopted when a heat pattern does not respond to medicinals bitter in flavor and cold in property since fever is caused by deficiency of kidney-yin.

诸气膹郁，皆属于肺［zhū qì fèn yù, jiē shǔ yú fèi］All qi disorders marked by short breath or oppression indicate problems of the lung.

诸湿肿满，皆属于脾［zhū shī zhǒng mǎn, jiē shǔ yú pí］All dampness diseases marked by swelling and fullness are ascribed to the spleen.

诸痛痒疮，皆属于心［zhū tòng yǎng chuāng, jiē shǔ yú xīn］All painful and itchy sores are ascribed to the heart.

诸阳之会［zhū yáng zhī huì］yang convergence 头者，～。The head is the site where all the yang meridians meet.

潴 zhū

潴留［zhū liú］retention 尿 ~ retention of urine

竹 zhú

竹罐［zhú guàn］bamboo cup

竹片固定［zhú piàn gù dìng］fixation with bamboo splints

竹枕［zhú zhěn］bamboo pillow

逐 zhú

逐水［zhú shuǐ］expelling retained water ~ 消肿 expelling retained water to relieve edema

逐瘀［zhú yū］expelling stagnated blood or blood stasis ~ 散结 expelling stagnated blood and disintegrating masses

主 zhǔ

主色［zhǔ sè］normal complexion

主食［zhǔ shí］staple food

主诉［zhǔ sù］complaint

主血脉［zhǔ xuè mài］governing blood and vessels

主治［zhǔ zhì］indication ~ 医师 attending doctor, doctor in charge

煮 zhǔ

煮药［zhǔ yào］decocting herbal medicinals

助 zhù

助阳［zhù yáng］reinforcing yang 温肾 ~ warming the kidney and reinforcing yang/ ~ 解表 reinforcing yang and releasing an exterior pattern

驻 zhù

驻颜［zhù yán］preserving youthful looks ~ 有术 possessing the secret of preserving youthful looks

祝 zhù

祝由［zhù yóu］pray-healing （incantation and talisman）

痒 zhù

痒夏［zhù xià］summer non-acclimatization

转篆 ZHUAN

转 zhuǎn

转胞［zhuǎn bāo］urinary bladder colic and pregnant dysuria colic

转基因［zhuǎn jī yīn］genetically modified ~ 食品 genetically modified food

转胯运腰［zhuǎn kuà yùn yāo］moving the hip and lower back

转膝［zhuǎn xī］rotating knees ~ 是一种练功方法。Rotating knees is a *qigong* exercise.

篆 zhuàn

篆刻［zhuàn kè］seal carving (cutting) ~ 养性法 cultivating one's character with seal carving. / ~ 是一种源于中国的传统的艺术形式。Seal cutting is a traditional art form originating in China.

壮 ZHUANG

壮 zhuàng

壮［zhuàng］moxa-cone；vigorous ~ 火 vigorous fire, hyperactive yang-qi/灸

Z

一 ~ moxibustion with one moxa-cone

壮火食气［zhuàng huǒ shí qì］original qi encroached by hyperactive yang-qi

壮热［zhuàng rè］high fever ~ 不止 persistent high fever

壮阳［zhuàng yáng］invigorating yang ~ 之品易伤正气。 Medicinals that invigorate yang are predisposed to impairment of healthy qi.

壮医学［zhuàng yī xué］Zhuang ethnic medicine

灼浊着 ZHUO

灼 zhuó

灼热［zhuó rè］high fever；burning 胃脘 ~ burning sensation in the stomach

灼痛［zhuó tòng］burning pain

浊 zhuó

浊［zhuó］turbid；unusable

着 zhuó

着痹［zhuó bì］arthralgia due to dampness

滋资子紫自 ZI

滋 zī

滋补［zī bǔ］nourishing，tonifying ~ 肝肾 tonifying the liver and kidney／~ 气血 building up qi and blood／~ 食品 nutritive food

滋补肾精［zī bǔ shèn jīng］replenishing kidney-essence ~ 治疗腰膝酸软。 Weakness and aching pain of the lower back and knees are treated by replenishing the kidney-essence.

滋水涵木［zī shuǐ hán mù］nourishing water phase（kidney）and wood phase（liver）

滋养［zī yǎng］·nourishing ~ 品 nutriment

资 zī

资气者食［zī qì zhě shí］ qi supplemented by food 主身者神，养气者精，益精者气，~。 The body is dominated by spirit and qi is nourished by essence. Essence boosting relies on qi and qi is supplemented by food.

子 zǐ

子病及母［zǐ bìng jí mǔ］disorder of a child-organ affecting the mother-organ

子烦［zǐ fán］restlessness during pregnancy

子宫［zǐ gōng］uterus, womb

子午觉［zǐ wǔ jiào］midnight sleep, midday nap

子午流注［zǐ wǔ liú zhù］midnight-noon ebb flow

子喑［zǐ yīn］aphasia during pregnancy

紫 zǐ

紫癜［zǐ diān］purpura

紫舌［zǐ shé］purple tongue

自 zì

自汗［zì hàn］spontaneous sweating 气虚 ~ spontaneous sweating due to qi deficiency

自强不息［zì qiáng bù xī］making unremitting efforts to improve oneself

~的民族精神 the national spirit of constantly striving for becoming stronger/天行健, 君子以 ~。The operation of nature is vigorous, and men work hard to improve themselves.

自然规律[zì rán guī lù] law of nature 遵循 ~ following the law of nature

自然呼吸 [zì rán hū xī] natural respiration, general breathing ~ 状态 in natural respiration/练功前应放松身体, 保持 ~。Before *qigong* exercise, one should relax all over and do natural respiration.

自然死亡[zì rán sǐ wáng] natural death

自然主义[zì rán zhǔ yì] naturalism

自我暗示[zì wǒ àn shì] self-suggestion

自信[zì xìn] being confident

自寻烦恼[zì xún fán nǎo] worrying oneself needlessly

自由自在[zì yóu zì zài] leisurely and carefree

自怨自艾[zì yuàn zì yì] full of remorse and self-reproach 何必 ~ 呢? Why are you still reproaching yourself about things?

自知之明[zì zhī zhī míng] wisdom of self-knowledge 人贵有 ~。Self-knowledge is wisdom.

自足[zì zú] self-satisfied 自给 ~ being self-supporting and self-sufficient

宗 ZONG
宗 zōng

宗筋[zōng jīn] all tendons; penis and testes

宗脉[zōng mài] convergence of meridians

宗气[zōng qì] pectoral qi ~ 泄 leakage of pectoral qi/ ~ 不足 lack of pectoral qi

走 ZOU
走 zǒu

走方医[zǒu fāng yī] itinerant healer

走罐法[zǒu guàn fǎ] sliding cupping

走味儿[zǒu wèi er] losing flavor

足阻 ZU
足 zú

足部反射[zú bù fǎn shè] foot reflection

足要常搓[zú yào cháng cuō] rubbing the sole center often ~ , 腹要常摩。Rub the sole center often and apply massage to the abdomen frequently.

足浴[zú yù] foot bath ~ 可以促进人体脚部血液循环, 达到改善脚部经络, 促进人体健康的目的。Foot bath promotes foot blood circulation to boost the meridian function and to improve health.

阻 zǔ

阻力运动[zǔ lì yùn dòng] resistance movement

醉 ZUI
醉 zuì

醉以入房[zuì yǐ rù fáng] having sexual

Z

activity after getting drunk

佐坐 ZUO

佐 zuǒ

佐餐服食［zuǒ cān fú shí］going with rice or bread

佐药［zuǒ yào］assistant medicinal ~ 的作用是配合辅助君、臣药更好地发挥作用,同时佐制其毒性作用。The assistant medicinals in a prescription work to help strengthen the action of the chief, deputy medicinals and relieve the toxic and side effect.

坐 zuò

坐北朝(向)南［zuò běi cháo（xiàng）nán］facing south 卧室的方向以 ~ 为佳。It is better for a bedroom to face south.

坐禅［zuò chán］meditation

坐式［zuò shì］sitting posture 太极拳半 ~ half sitting posture in tai chi chuan

坐忘［zuò wàng］sitting in oblivion; sitting and forgetting oneself and the world around 安心 ~ sitting in oblivion with pacified mind/~ 心斋 sitting in oblivion and purifying the mind

坐浴［zuò yù］hip bath

Z

汉字笔画索引

四 画

五　画

六　画

七　画

八　画

九 画

十一画

十二画

十四画

十六画

十七画

附录

养生相关典籍
Ancient Classics Related to Health Preservation

B

《抱朴子内篇》*Bao Pu Zi Nei Pian*
（*Bao Pu Zi*, Vol. I）

《保婴撮要》*Bao Ying Cuo Yao*
（*Essentials of the Care of Infants*）

《备急千金要方》*Bei Ji Qian Jin Yao Fang*（*Important Prescriptions Worth a Thousand Pieces of Gold for Emergency*）

《本草纲目》*Ben Cao Gang Mu*
（*Compendium of Materia Medica*）

《本草纲目拾遗》*Ben Cao Gang Mu Shi Yi*（*Supplement to the Compendium of Materia Medica*）

《本草蒙筌》*Ben Cao Meng Quan*
（*Enlightening Primer of Materia Medica*）

《本草拾遗》*Ben Cao Shi Yi*
（*Supplement to the Materia Medica*）

《濒湖脉学》*Bin Hu Mai Xue*（*Binhu's Sphygmology*）

D

《滇南本草》*Dian Nan Ben Cao*
（*Materia Medica of South Yunnan*）

《东坡养生集》*Dong Po Yang Sheng Ji*
（*Su Dongpo's Manual for Fitness*）

F

《傅青主女科》*Fu Qing Zhu Nü Ke*（*Fu Qingzhu's Obstetrics and Gynecology*）

H

《黄帝内经》*Huang Di Nei Jing*
（*Huangdi's Canon of Medicine*）

《黄帝内经太素》*Huang Di Nei Jing Tai Su*（*Great Simplicity of Huangdi's Canon of Medicine*）

J

《金匮要略》*Jin Gui Yao Lüe*（*Synopsis of the Golden Chamber*）

《经效产宝》*Jing Xiao Chan Bao*
（*Valuable Experience in Obstetrics*）

《景岳全书》*Jing Yue Quan Shu*
（*Jingyue's Complete Works*）

《救荒本草》*Jiu Huang Ben Cao*
（*Materia Medica for Famine Relief*）

L

《兰室秘藏》*Lan Shi Mi Cang*（*Secret*

Book of the Orchid Chamber)

《老老恒言》Lao Lao Heng Yan (Common Saying for the Aged)

《雷公炮炙论》Lei Gong Pao Zhi Lun (Master Lei's Discourse on Medicinal Processing)

《类经》Lei Jing(Classified Classic)

《类经附翼》Lei Jing Fu Yi(Appendices to the Classified Classic)

《灵枢》Ling Shu(Miraculous Pivot)

《陆地仙经》Lu Di Xian Jing (Annotation to Daoyin Exercise)

M

《脉经》Mai Jing(Pulse Classic)

《梦溪笔谈》Meng Xi Bi Tan(Dream Pool Essays)

N

《难经》Nan Jing(Classic of Difficult Issues)

P

《脾胃论》Pi Wei Lun(Treatise on the Spleen and Stomach)

Q

《千金翼方》Qian Jin Yi Fang (Supplement to the Prescriptions Worth a Thousand Pieces of Gold for Emergency)

R

《儒门事亲》Ru Men Shi Qin (Confucian's Duties to Parents)

S

《山家清供》Shan Jia Qing Gong (Cook Book of Quanzhou)

《伤寒论》Shang Han Lun(Treatise on Cold-induced Diseases)

《摄生总要》She Sheng Zong Yao(The Essentials of Preserving Health)

《神农本草经》Shen Nong Ben Cao Jing (Shen Nong's Herbal Classic)

《食疗本草》Shi Liao Ben Cao(Herbals in Dietary Therapy)

《食物本草》Shi Wu Ben Cao(Herbals as Food)

《寿世保元》Shou Shi Bao Yuan (Longevity and Life Preservation)

《寿世青编》Shou Shi Qing Bian (Collected Records for Prolonging Life)

《素问》Su Wen(Plain Questions)

《素问病机气宜保命集》Su Wen Bing Ji Qi Yi Bao Ming Ji(Collection of Writings on the Mechanism of Disease, Qi Regulation and Safeguard of Life Discussed in the Plain Questions)

《素问玄机原病式》Su Wen Xuan Ji Yuan Bing Shi (Explanation to Mysterious Pathogenesis and Etiology Based on the Plain Questions)

《随息居饮食谱》Sui Xi Ju Yin Shi Pu (Food and Drink Recipes from the Lay Buddhist Sui-Xi)

T

《太平惠民和剂局方》*Tai Ping Hui Min He Ji Ju Fang*(*Formulary of the Bureau of Taiping People's Welfare Pharmacy*)

《太平圣惠方》*Tai Ping Sheng Hui Fang*(*Taiping Holy Prescriptions for Universal Relief*)

《唐本草》*Tang Ben Cao*(*Materia Medica of the Tang Dynasty*)

W

《外台秘要》*Wai Tai Mi Yao*(*Arcane Essentials from the Imperial Library*)

《万病回春》*Wan Bing Hui Chun*(*Restoration of Health from Diseases*)

《卫生宝鉴》*Wei Sheng Bao Jian*(*Precious Mirror of Hygiene*)

《五十二病方》*Wu Shi Er Bing Fang*(*Prescriptions for Fifty-two Diseases*)

X

《先醒斋医学广笔记》*Xian Xing Zhai Yi Xue Guang Bi Ji*(*Extensive Notes on Medicine from Xian Xing Studio*)

《小儿药证直诀》*Xiao Er Yao Zheng Zhi Jue*(*Key to the Theraputics of Children's Diseases*)

《新修本草》*Xin Xiu Ben Cao*(*Newly Revised Materia Medica*)

Y

《养老奉亲书》*Yang Lao Feng Qin Shu*(*On Providing for the Aged and Taking Good Care of Parents*)

《养生类纂》*Yang Sheng Lei Zuan*(*Categorized Compilations of Health Preservation*)

《养生三要》*Yang Sheng San Yao*(*Three Essentials in Health Preservation*)

《养性延命录》*Yang Xing Yan Ming Lu*(*Recordings of the Healing Art for Health and Health Preservation*)

《医贯》*Yi Guan*(*Key Link of Medicine*)

《易筋经》*Yi Jin Jing*(*Muscle-bone Strengthening Exercise*)

《颐养编》*Yi Yang Bian*(*Compiled Texts on Keeping Fit*)

《医宗金鉴》*Yi Zong Jin Jian*(*The Golden Mirror of Medicine*)

《饮膳正要》*Yin Shan Zheng Yao*(*Principles of Correct Diet*)

《幼幼集成》*You You Ji Cheng*(*Complete Works on Children's Diseases*)

《幼幼新书》*You You Xin Shu*(*New Book on Pediatrics*)

Z

《针灸大成》*Zhen Jiu Da Cheng*(*Great Compendium of Acupuncture and Moxibustion*)

《针灸大全》*Zhen Jiu Da Quan*(*Great

Complete Collection of Acupuncture and Moxibustion)

《针灸甲乙经》*Zhen Jiu Jia Yi Jing* (*ABC Classic of Acupuncture and Moxibustion*)

《珍珠囊》*Zhen Zhu Nang* (*Pouch of Pearls*)

《周易参同契》*Zhou Yi Can Tong Qi* (*The Kinship of The Three, According to The Book of Changes*)

《肘后备急方》*Zhou Hou Bei Ji Fang* (*Handbook of Prescriptions for Emergency*)

《中华本草》*Zhong Hua Ben Cao* (*Chinese Materia Medica*)

《诸病源候论》*Zhu Bing Yuan Hou Lun* (*Treatise on Causes and Manifestations of Various Diseases*)

《遵生八笺》*Zun Sheng Ba Jian* (*Eight Essential Chapters on Conforming to Life*)

养生相关中药

Chinese Medcinals Applied to Health Preservation

食药物质名单
Food Materials with Dual-purpose of Medicine and Food

中药名称	汉语拼音	英文名称	拉丁文名
八角茴香	Bājiǎohuíxiāng	Chinese Star Anise	*Anisi Stellati Fructus*
白扁豆	Báibiǎndòu	White Hyacinth Bean	*Lablab Semen Album*
白扁豆花	Báibiǎndòuhuā	White Hyacinth Bean Flower	*Lablab Flos Album*
白果	Báiguǒ	Ginkgo Seed	*Ginkgo Semen*
百合	Bǎihé	Lily Bulb	*Lilii Bulbus*
白茅根	Báimáogēn	Lalang Grass Rhizome	*Imperatae Rhizoma*
白芷	Báizhǐ	Dahurian Angelica Root	*Angelicae Dahuricae Radix*
薄荷	Bòhe	Peppermint	*Menthae Haplocalycis Herba*
荜茇	Bìbó	Long Pepper	*Piperis Longui Fructus*
布渣叶	Bùzhāyè	Paniculate Microcos Leaf	*Microctis Folium*
草果	Cǎoguǒ	Tsaoko Fruit	*Tsaoko Fructus*
陈皮	Chénpí	DriedTangerine Peel	*Citri Reticulatae Pericarpium*
赤小豆	Chìxiǎodòu	Rice Bean	*Vignae Semen*
大枣	Dàzǎo	Chinese Date	*Jujubae Fructus*
淡豆豉	Dàndòuchǐ	Fermented Soybean	*Sojae Semen Praeparatum*
淡竹叶	Dànzhúyè	Lophatherum Herb	*Lophatheri Herba*
当归	Dāngguī	Chinese Angelica	*Angelicae Sinensis Radix*
刀豆	Dāodòu	Jack Bean	*Canavaliae Semen*
丁香	Dīngxiāng	Clove	*Caryophylli Flos*
阿胶	Ējiāo	Donkey-hide Glue	*Asini Corii Colla*
榧子	Fěizi	Grand Torreya Seed	*Torreyae Semen*
粉葛	Fěngě	Thomson Kudzuvine Root	*Puerariae Thomsonii Radix*
蜂蜜	Fēngmì	Honey	*Mel*

中药名称	汉语拼音	英文名称	拉丁文名
佛手	Fóshǒu	Finger Citron	*Citri Sarcodactylis Fructus*
茯苓	Fúlíng	IndianBread	*Poria*
覆盆子	Fùpénzǐ	Palmleaf Raspberry Fruit	*Rubi Fructus*
甘草	Gāncǎo	Liquorice Root	*Glycyrrhizae Radix et Rhizoma*
干姜	Gānjiāng	Zingiber(Dried Ginger)	*Zingiberis Rhizoma*
高良姜	Gāoliángjiāng	Lesser Galangal Rhizome	*Alpiniae Officinarum Rhizoma*
葛根	Gěgēn	Kudzuvine Root	*Puerariae Lobatae Radix*
枸杞子	Gǒuqǐzǐ	Barbary Wolfberry Fruit	*Lycii Fructus*
荷叶	Héyè	LotusLeaf	*Nelumbinis Folium*
黑胡椒	Hēihújiāo	Pepper Fruit	*Piper Nigrum*
黑芝麻	Hēizhīma	Black Sesame	*Sesami Semen Nigrum*
花椒	Huājiāo	Pricklyash Peel	*Zanthoxyli Pericarpium*
槐花	Huáihuā	Pagodatree Flower	*Sophorae Flos*
黄精	Huángjīng	Solomonseal Rhizome	*Polygonati Rhizoma*
火麻仁	Huǒmárén	Hemp Seed	*Cannabis Fructus*
藿香	Huòxiāng	Cablin Patchouli Herb	*Pogostemonis Herba*
鸡内金	Jīnèijīn	Chicken's Gizzard-skin	*Galli Gigerii Endothelium Corneum*
姜黄	Jiānghuáng	Turmeric	*Curcumae Longae Rhizoma*
桔梗	Jiégěng	Platycodon Root	*Platycodonis Radix*
金银花	Jīnyínhuā	Japanese Honeysuckle Flower	*Lonicerae Japonicae Flos*
橘红	Júhóng	Red Tangerine Peel	*Citri Exocarpium Rubrum*
菊花	Júhuā	Chrysanthemum Flower	*Chrysanthemi Flos*
菊苣	Jújù	Chicory Herb	*Cichorii Herba Cichorii Radix*
决明子	Juémíngzǐ	Cassia Seed	*Cassiae Semen*
苦杏仁	Kǔxìngrén	Bitter Apricot Seed	*Armeniacae Semen Amarum*
昆布	Kūnbù	Kelp or Tangle	*Laminariae Thallus*
莱菔子	Láifúzǐ	Radish Seed	*Raphani Semen*
莲子	Liánzǐ	Lotus Seed	*Nelumbinis Semen*
灵芝	Língzhī	Glossy Ganoderma	*Ganoderma*

续表

中药名称	汉语拼音	英文名称	拉丁文名
龙眼肉	Lóngyǎnròu	Longan Aril	*Longan Arillus*
芦根	Lúgēn	Reed Rhizome	*Phragmitis Rhizoma*
罗汉果	Luóhànguǒ	Grosvenor Momordica Fruit	*Siraitiae Fructus*
马齿苋	Mǎchǐxiàn	Purslane Herb	*Portulacae Herba*
麦芽	Màiyá	Germinated Barley	*Hordei Fructus Germinatus*
玫瑰花	Méiguīhuā	Rose Flower	*Rosae Rugosae Flos*
牡蛎	Mǔlì	Oyster Shell	*Ostreae Concha*
木瓜	Mùguā	Common Floweringqince Fruit	*Chaenomelis Fructus*
胖大海	Pàngdàhǎi	Boat-fruited Sterculia Seed	*Sterculiae Lychnophorae Semen*
蒲公英	Púgōngyīng	Dandelion	*Taraxaci Herba*
蕲蛇	Qíshé	Long-nosed Pit Viper	*Agkistrodon*
芡实	Qiànshí	Gordon Euryale Seed	*Euryales Semen*
青果	Qīngguǒ	Chinese White Olive	*Canarii Fructus*
人参	Rénshēn	Ginseng	*Ginseng Radix et Rhizoma*
肉苁蓉	Ròucōngróng	Desertliving Cistanche	*Cistanches Herba*
肉豆蔻	Ròudòukòu	Nutmeg	*Myristicae Semen*
肉桂	Ròuguì	Cassia Bark	*Cinnamomi Cortex*
桑椹	Sāngshèn	Mulberry Fruit	*Mori Fructus*
桑叶	Sāngyè	Mulberry Leaf	*Mori Folium*
沙棘	Shājí	Seabuckthorn Fruit	*Hippophae Fructus*
砂仁	Shārén	Villous Amomum Fruit	*Amomi Fructus*
山柰	Shānnài	Galanga Resurrectionlily Rhizome	*Kaempferiae Rhizoma*
山药	Shānyào	CommonYam Rhizome	*Dioscoreae Rhizoma*
山银花	Shānyínhuā	Honeysuckle Flower	*Lonicerae Flos*
山楂	Shānzhā	Hawthorn Fruit	*Crataegi Fructus*
生姜	Shēngjiāng	Fresh Ginger	*Zingiberis Rhizoma Recens*
松花粉	Sōnghuāfěn	Pine Pollen	*Pini Pollen*
酸枣仁	Suānzǎorén	Spine Date Seed	*Ziziphi Spinosae Semen*
桃仁	Táorén	Peach Seed	*Persicae Semen*

续表

中药名称	汉语拼音	英文名称	拉丁文名
乌梅	Wūméi	Smoked Plum	*Mume Fructus*
乌梢蛇	Wūshāoshé	Black-tail Snake	*Zaocys*
西红花	Xīhónghuā	Saffron	*Croci Stigma*
夏枯草	Xiàkūcǎo	Common Selfheal Fruit-Spike	*Prunellae Spica*
香薷	Xiāngrú	Chinese Mosla	*Moslae Herba*
香橼	Xiāngyuán	Citron Fruit	*Citri Fructus*
小茴香	Xiǎohuíxiāng	Fennel	*Foeniculi Fructus*
小蓟	Xiǎojì	Field Thistle Herb	*Cirsii Herba*
薤白	Xièbái	Longstamen Onion Bulb	*Allii Macrostemonis Bulbus*
芫荽	Yánsuī	Chinese Parsley	*Coriandri Herba*
薏苡仁	Yìyǐrén	Coix seed	*Coicis Semen*
益智仁	Yìzhìrén	Sharpleaf Glangal Fruit	*Alpniae Oxyphyllae Fructus*
余甘子	Yúgānzǐ	Emblic Leaffower Fruit	*Phyllanthi Fructus*
郁李仁	Yùlǐrén	Chinese Dwarf Cherry Seed	*Pruni Semen*
鱼腥草	Yúxīngcǎo	Heartleaf Houttuynia Herb	*Houttuyniae Herba*
玉竹	Yùzhú	Fragrant Solomonseal Rhizome	*Polygonati Odorati Rhizoma*
枳椇子	Zhǐjǔzǐ	Hovenia dulcis	*Hoveniae Semen*
紫苏	Zǐsū	Perilla Leaf and Stem	*Perillae Folium et Caulis*
紫苏子	Zǐsūzǐ	Perilla Fruit	*Perillae Fructus*

可用于保健食品的物品名单
Food Materials That Can be Applied to Health Food

中药名称	汉语拼音	英文名称	拉丁文名
巴戟天	Bājǐtiān	Morinda Root	*Morindae Officinalis Radix*
白豆蔻	Báidòukòu	Round Cardamon Fruit	*Amomi Fructus Rotundus*
白及	Báijí	Common Bletilla Tuber	*Bletillae Rhizoma*
白芍	Báisháo	White Peony Root	*Paeoniae Radix Alba*
白术	Báizhú	Largehead Atractylodes Rhizome	*Atractylodis Macrocephalae Rhizoma*
柏子仁	Bǎizǐrén	Chinese Arborvitae Kernel	*Platycladi Semen*
北沙参	Běishāshēn	Coastal Glehnia Root	*Glehniae Radix*

续表

中药名称	汉语拼音	英文名称	拉丁文名
荜茇	Bìbó	Long Pepper	*Piperis Lonui Fructus*
鳖甲	Biējiǎ	Turtle Carapace	*Trionycis Carapax*
补骨脂	Bǔgǔzhǐ	Malaytea Scurfpea Fruit	*Psoraleae Fructus*
苍术	Cāngzhú	Atractylodes Rhizome	*Atractylodis Rhizoma*
侧柏叶	Cèbǎiyè	Chinese Arborvitae Twig and Leaf	*Platycladi Cacumen*
车前草	Chēqiáncǎo	Plantain Herb	*Plantaginis Herba*
车前子	Chēqiánzǐ	Plantain Seed	*Plantaginis Semen*
赤芍	Chìsháo	Red Peony Root	*Paeoniae Radix Rubra*
川贝母	Chuānbèimǔ	Tendrilleaf Fritillary Bulb	*Fritillariae Cirrhosae Bulbus*
川牛膝	Chuānniúxī	Medicinal Cyathula Root	*Cyathulae Radix*
川芎	Chuānxiōng	Szechwan Lovage Rhizome	*Chuanxiong Rhizoma*
刺五加	Cìwǔjiā	Manyprickle Acanthopanax	*Acanthopanacis Senticosi Radix et Rhizoma seu Caulis*
大蓟	Dàjì	Japanese Thistle Herb	*Cirsii Japonici Herba*
丹参	Dānshēn	Danshen Root	*Salviae Miltiorrhizae Radix et Rhizoma*
当归	Dāngguī	Chinese Angelica	*Angelicae Sinensis Radix*
党参	Dǎngshēn	Tangshen	*Codonopsis Radix*
地骨皮	Dìgǔpí	Chinese Wolfberry Root-bark	*Lycii Cortex*
杜仲	Dùzhòng	Eucommia Bark	*Eucommiae Cortex*
杜仲叶	Dùzhòngyè	Eucommia Leaf	*Eucommiae Folium*
番泻叶	Fānxièyè	Senna Leaf	*Sennae Folium*
蜂胶	Fēngjiāo	Propolis	*Propolis*
蛤蚧	Géjiè	Tokay Gecko	*Gecko*
骨碎补	Gǔsuìbǔ	Fortune's Drynaria Rhizome	*Drynariae Rhizoma*
龟甲	Guījiǎ	Tortoise Carapace and Plastron	*Testudinis Carapax et Plastrum*
诃子	Hēzǐ	Medicine Terminalia Fruit	*Chebulae Fructus*
红花	Hónghuā	Safflower	*Carthami Flos*
红景天	Hóngjǐngtiān	Bigflower Rhodiola Root	*Rhodiolae Crenulatae Radix et Rhizoma*

中药名称	汉语拼音	英文名称	拉丁文名
厚朴	Hòupò	Officinal Magnolia Bark	*Magnoliae Officinalis Cortex*
厚朴花	Hòupòhuā	Officinal Magnolia Flower	*Magnoliae Officinalis Flos*
湖北贝母	Húběibèimǔ	Hupeh Fritillary Bulb	*Fritillariae Hupehensis Bulbus*
槐角	Huáijiǎo	Japanese Pagodatree Pod	*Sophorae Fructus*
怀牛膝	Huáiniúxī	Twotoothed Achyranthes Root	*Achyranthis Bidentatae Radix*
黄芪	Huángqí	Milkvetch Root	*Astragali Radix*
积雪草	Jīxuěcǎo	Asiatic Pennywort Herb	*Centellae Herba*
蒺藜	Jíli	Puncturevine Caltrop Fruit	*Tribuli Fructus*
姜黄	Jiānghuáng	Turmeric	*Curcumae Longae Rhizoma*
金荞麦	Jīnqiáomài	Golden Buckwheat Rhizome	*Fagopyri Dibotryis Rhizoma*
金樱子	Jīnyīngzǐ	Cherokee Rose Fruit	*Rosae Laevigatae Fructus*
韭菜子	Jiǔcàizǐ	Tuber Onion Seed	*Allii Tuberosi Semen*
苦丁茶	Kǔdīngchá	Immature Chinese Holly Leaf	*Ilicis Cornutae Folium*
芦荟	Lúhùi	Aloes	*Aloe*
罗布麻	Luóbùmá	Dogbane Leaf	*Apocyni Veneti Folium*
马鹿茸	Mǎlùróng	Pilose Antler	*Cervi Cornu Pantotrichum*
麦门冬	Màiméndōng	Dwarf Lilyturf Tuber	*Ophiopogonis Radix*
玫瑰花	Méiguihuā	Rose Flower	*Rosae Rugosae Flos*
玫瑰茄	Méiguiqié	Roselle Calyx	*Hibiscus Sabdariffa*
墨旱莲	Mòhànlián	Yerbadetajo Herb	*Ecliptae Herba*
牡丹皮	Mǔdānpí	Tree Peony Bark	*Moutan Cortex*
木香	Mùxiāng	Common Aucklandia Root	*Aucklandiae Radix*
木贼	Mùzéi	Common Scouring Rush Herb	*Equiseti Hiemalis Herba*
牛蒡子	Niúbàngzǐ	Great Burdock Achene	*Arctii Fructus*
女贞子	Nǚzhēnzǐ	Glossy Privet Fruit	*Ligustri Lucidi Fructus*
佩兰	Pèilán	Fortune Eupatorium Herb	*Eupatorii Herba*
平贝母	Píngbèimǔ	Ussuri Fritillary Bulb	*Fritillariae Ussuriensis Bulbus*
蒲黄	Púhuáng	Cattail Pollen	*Typhae Pollen*
茜草	Qiàncǎo	Indian Madder Root	*Rubiae Radix et Rhizoma*

中药名称	汉语拼音	英文名称	拉丁文名
青皮	Qīngpí	Green Tangerine Peel	*Citri Reticulatae PericarpiumViride*
人参	Rénshēn	Ginseng	*Ginseng Radix et Rhizoma*
人参叶	Rénshēnyè	Ginseng Leaf	*Ginseng Folium*
三七	Sānqī	Sanchi	*Notoginseng Radix et Rhizoma*
桑白皮	Sāngbáipí	White Mulberry Root-bark	*Mori Cortex*
桑枝	Sāngzhī	Mulberry Twig	*Mori Ramulus*
沙苑子	Shāyuànzǐ	Flatstem Milkvetch Seed	*Astragali Complanati Semen*
山茱萸	Shānzhūyú	Asiatic Cornelian Cherry Fruit	*Corni Fructus*
升麻	Shēngmá	Largetrifoliolious Bugbane Rhizome	*Cimicifugae Rhizoma*
生地黄	Shēngdìhuáng	Rehmannia Root	*Rehmanniae Radix*
生何首乌	Shēnghéshǒuwū	Fleeceflower Root	*Polygoni Multiflori Radix*
石斛	Shíhú	Dendrobium	*Dendrobii Caulis*
石决明	Shíjuémíng	Abalone Shell	*Haliotidis Concha*
首乌藤	Shǒuwūténg	Tuber Fleeceflower Stem	*Polygoni Multiflori Caulis*
熟地黄	Shúdìhuáng	Prepared Rehmannia Root	*Rehmanniae Radix Praeparata*
太子参	Tàizǐshēn	Heterophylly Falsestarwort Root	*Pseudostellariae Radix*
天麻	Tiānmá	Tall Gastrodia Tuber	*Gastrodiae Rhizoma*
天门冬	Tiānméndōng	Cochinchinese Asparagus Root	*Asparagi Radix*
土茯苓	Tǔfúlíng	Glabrous Greenbrier Rhizome	*Smilacis Glabrae Rhizoma*
菟丝子	Tùsīzǐ	Dodder Seed	*Cuscutae Semen*
五加皮	Wǔjiāpí	Slenderstyle Acanthopanax Bark	*Acanthopanacis Cortex*
五味子	Wǔwèizǐ	Chinese Magnoliavine Fruit	*Schisandrae Chinensis Fructus*
吴茱萸	Wúzhūyú	Medicinal Euodia Fruit	*Euodiae Fructus*
西洋参	Xīyángshēn	American Ginseng	*Panacis Quinquefolii Radix*
香附	Xiāngfù	Nutgrass Galingale Rhizome	*Cyperi Rhizoma*
玄参	Xuánshēn	Figwort Root	*Scrophulariae Radix*
野菊花	Yějúhuā	Wild Chrysanthemum Flower	*Chrysanthemi Indici Flos*
益母草	Yìmǔcǎo	Motherwort Herb	*Leonuri Herba*

续表

中药名称	汉语拼音	英文名称	拉丁文名
银杏叶	Yínxìngyè	Ginkgo Leaf	*Ginkgo Folium*
淫羊藿	Yínyánghuò	Epimedium Leaf	*Epimedii Folium*
远志	Yuǎnzhì	Thinleaf Milkwort Root	*Polygalae Radix*
泽兰	Zélán	Hirsute Shiny Bugleweed Herb	*Lycopi Herba*
泽泻	Zéxiè	Oriental Waterplantain Rhizome	*Alismatis Rhizoma*
浙贝母	Zhèbèimǔ	Thunberg Fritillary Bulb	*Fritillariae Thunbergii Bulbus*
珍珠	Zhēnzhū	Pearl	*Margarita*
制何首乌	Zhìhéshǒuwū	Prepared Fleeceflower Root	*Polygoni Multiflori Radix Praeparata*
知母	Zhīmǔ	Common Anemarrhena Rhizome	*Anemarrhenae Rhizoma*
枳壳	Zhǐqiào	Orange Fruit	*Aurantii Fructus*
枳实	Zhǐshí	Immature Orange Fruit	*Aurantii Fructus Immaturus*
竹茹	Zhúrú	Bamboo Shavings	*Bambusae Caulis in Taenias*

保健食品禁用物品名单
Forbidden Materials in Health Food

中药名称	汉语拼音	英文名称	拉丁文名
八角莲	Bājiǎolián	Sixangular Dysosma Rhizome	*Dysosmatis Rhizoma et Radix*
巴豆	Bādòu	Croton Fruit	*Crotonis Fructus*
草乌	Cǎowū	Kusnezoff Monkshood Root	*Aconiti Kusnezoffii Radix*
蟾酥	Chánsū	Toad Venom	*Bufonis Venenum*
川乌	Chuānwū	Common Monkshood Mother Root	*Aconiti Radix*
颠茄	Diānqié	Belladonna Herb	*Belladonnae Herba*
甘遂	Gānsuí	Gansui Root	*Kansui Radix*
关木通	Guānmùtōng	Manchurian Dutchmanspipe Stem	*Aristolochiae Manshuriensis Caulis*
广防己	Guǎngfángjǐ	Aristolochia Fangchi	*Cocculus Orbiculatus(L.)DC.*
河豚	Hétún	Globefish	*Tetraodontidae*
黄花夹竹桃	Huánghuājiāzhútáo	Thevetia Peruviana	*Semen Thevetiae Peruvianae*
夹竹桃	Jiāzhútáo	Oleander	*Nerium Indicum Mill.*
京大戟	Jīngdàjǐ	Peking Euphorbia Root	*Euphorbiae Pekinensis Radix*
昆明山海棠	Kūnmíngshān hǎitáng	Tripterygium Hypoglaucum Hutch	*Tripterygium Hypoglaucu (Lévl.) Hutchins.*

续表

中药名称	汉语拼音	英文名称	拉丁文名
雷公藤	Léigōngténg	Tripterygium Wilfordii	*Tripterygium Wilfordii Radix*
藜芦	Lílú	Black False Hellebore	*Veratri Radix et Rhizoma*
铃兰	Línglán	Lily-Of-The-Valley	*Convallaria majalis*
硫磺	Líuhuáng	Sulfur	*Sulfur*
六角莲	Lìujiǎolián	Sixangular Dysosma Rhizome	*Dysosma Pleiantha*
骆驼蓬	Luòtuopéng	Peganum Harmala	*Peganum Harmala*
马钱子	Mǎqiánzǐ	Nux Vomica	*Strychni Semen*
莽草	Mǎngcǎo	Shikimmi	*Illicium Lanceolatum*
闹羊花	Nàoyánghuā	Yellow Azalea Flower	*Rhododendri Mollis Flos*
农吉利	Nóngjílì	Crotalaria Sessiliflora	*Crotalaria Herba*
砒霜	Pīshuāng	Arsenic	*Arsenicum Arsenolite*
千金子	Qiānjīnzǐ	Caper Euphorbia Seed	*Euphorbiae Semen*
牵牛子	Qiānniúzǐ	Pharbitis Seed	*Pharbitidis Semen*
山莨菪	Shānlàngdàng	Scopolia Tangutica Maxim.	*Anisodus Tanguticus*
生白附子	Shēngbáifùzǐ	Giant Typhonium Rhizome	*Typhonii Rhizoma*
生半夏	Shēngbànxià	Pinellia Tuber	*Pinelliae Rhizoma*
生狼毒	Shēnglángdú	Bracteole-lacked Euphorbia Root	*Euphorbiae Ebracteolatae Radix*
生天南星	Shēngtiānnánxīng	Jackinthepulpit Tuber	*Arisaematis Rhizoma*
石蒜	Shísuàn	Lycoris Radiata	*Lycoris Radiata Bulbus*
天仙子	Tiānxiānzǐ	Henbane Seed	*Hyoscyami Semen*
香加皮	Xiāngjiāpí	Chinese Silkvine Root-bark	*Periplocae Cortex*
雄黄	Xiónghuáng	Realgar	*Realgar*
羊角拗	Yángjiǎoniù	Divaricate Strophanthus	*Semen Strophanthii Divaricati*
洋金花	Yángjīnhuā	Datura Flower	*Daturae flos*
罂粟壳	Yīngsùqiào	Poppy Capsule	*Papaveris pericarpium*
朱砂	Zhūshā	Cinnabar	*Cinnabaris*

参 考 文 献

[1] 张有寯,李梃,郑敏. 汉英中医辞海[M]. 太原:山西人民出版社,1994.

[2] 方廷钰,嵇波,吴青. 新汉英中医学词典[M]. 2 版. 北京:中国医药科技出版社,2013.

[3] 方廷钰,陈锋,都立澜. 中医英语 300 句[M]. 北京:中国医药科技出版社,2018.

[4] 谢竹藩,谢方. 新编汉英中医药分类词典[M]. 2 版. 北京:外文出版社,2019.

[5] 图娅,方廷钰. History and Philosophy of Chinese Medicine[M]. 北京:人民卫生出版社,2014.

[6] 李照国. 简明英汉黄帝内经词典[M]. 北京:人民卫生出版社,2011.

[7] World Health Organization Western Pacific Region. WHO International Standard Terminologies On Traditional Medicine In The Western Pacific Region[M]. Manila:World Health Organization,2007.

[8] W. B. Saunders Company. Dorland's Illustrated Medical Dictionary[M]. 北京:人民卫生出版社,2001.

[9] 国家药典委员会. 中华人民共和国药典(英文版)[M]. 北京:中国医药科技出版社,2015.

[10] 朱丽,于海江. 牛津外语社英汉汉英词典[M]. 北京:外语教学与研究出版社,2010.

[11] 张健. 当代新编汉英词典[M]. 上海:上海世界图书出版公司,2002.

[12] 霍恩比. 牛津高阶英汉双解词典[M]. 9 版. 北京:商务印书馆,2018.

[13] 危东亚. 汉英词典(修订版)[M]. 北京:外语教学与研究出版社,1995.